Muscular Dystrophy - Research Updates and Therapeutic Strategies

Edited by Gisela Gaina

Published in London, United Kingdom

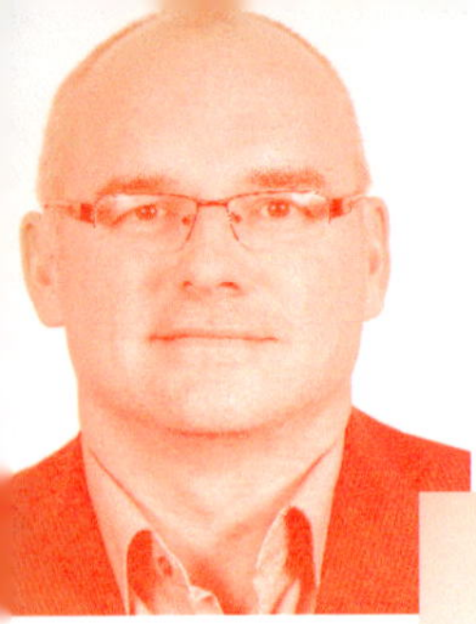
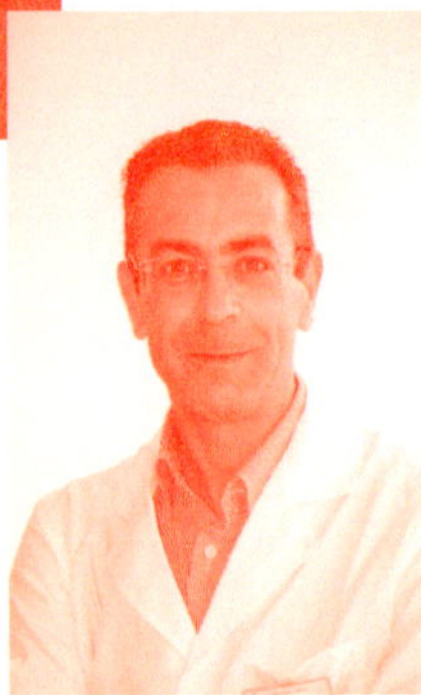
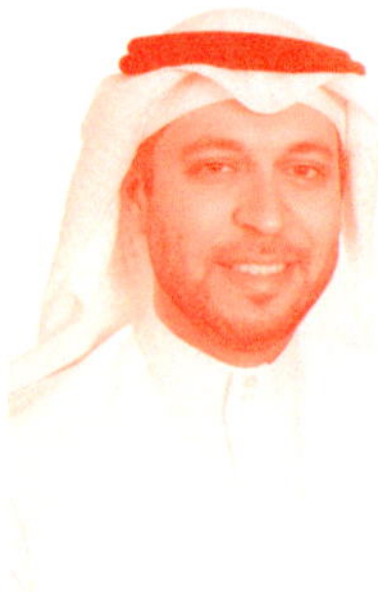
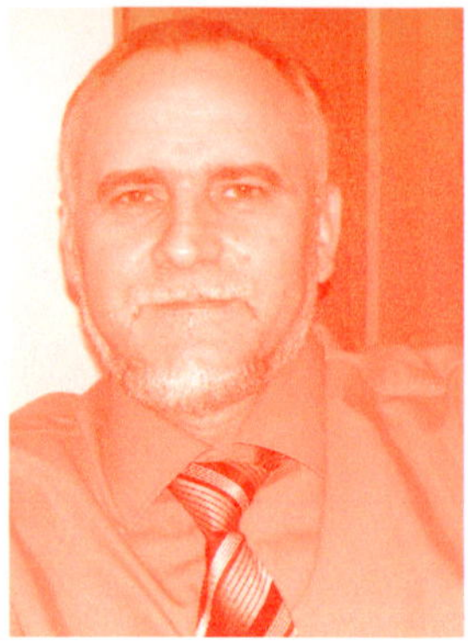
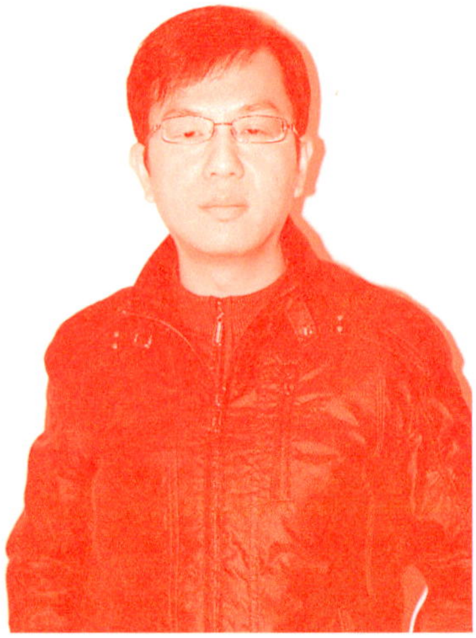
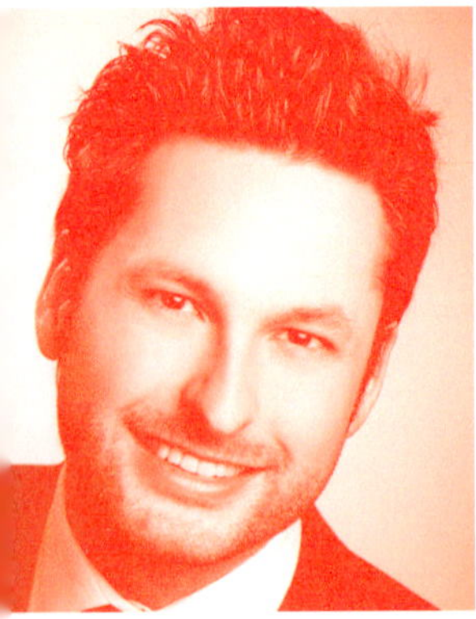
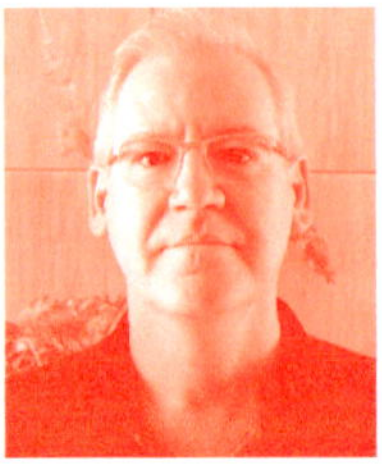

IntechOpen

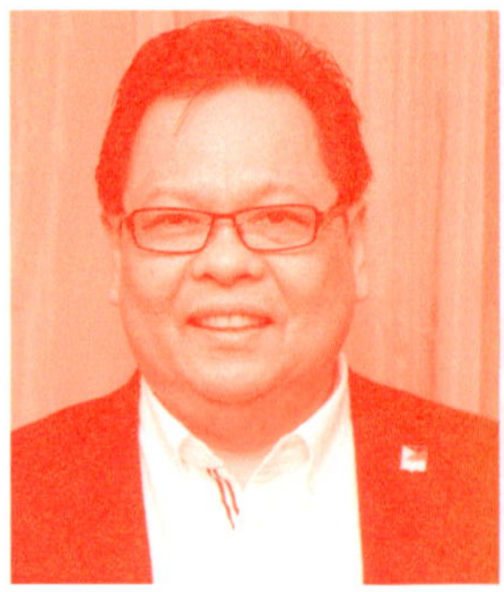
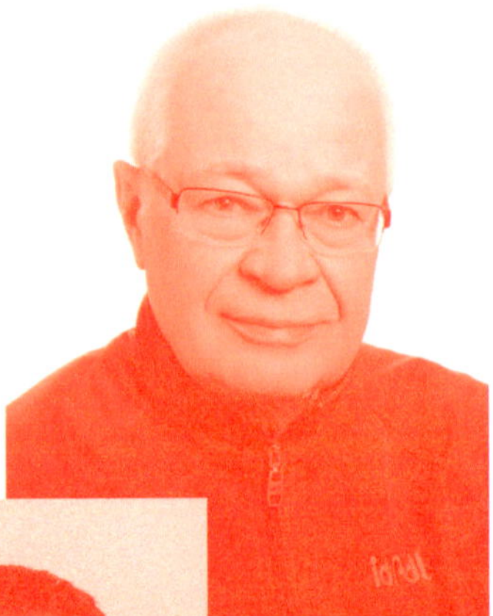
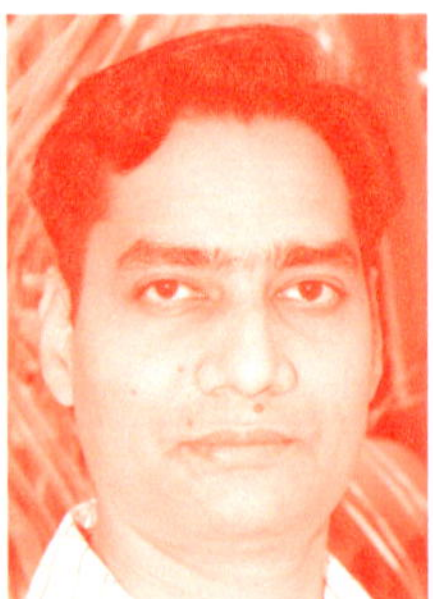
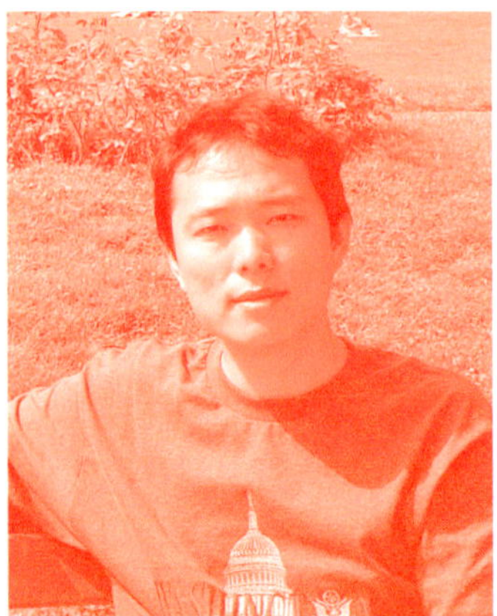
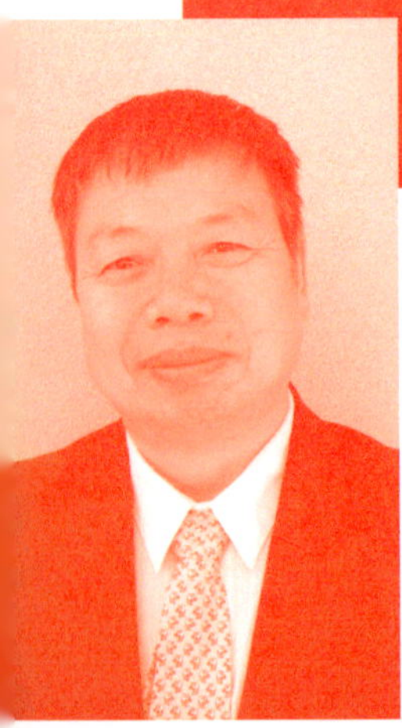
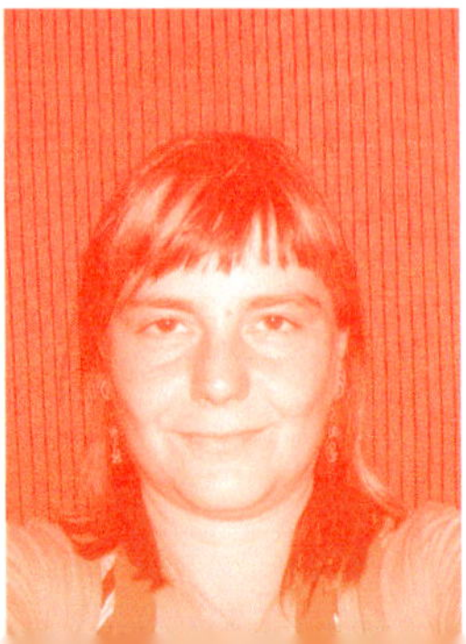

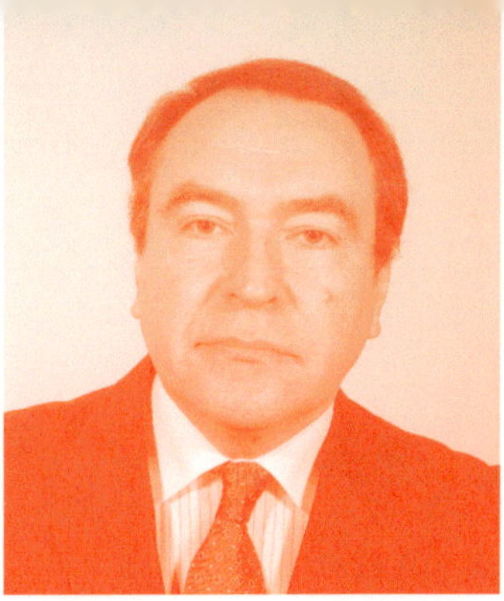
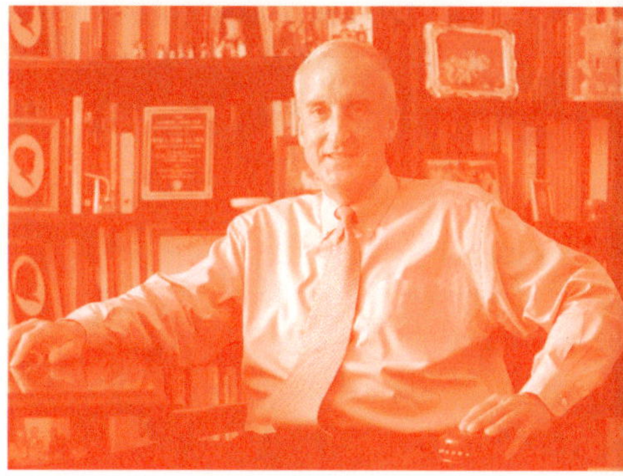
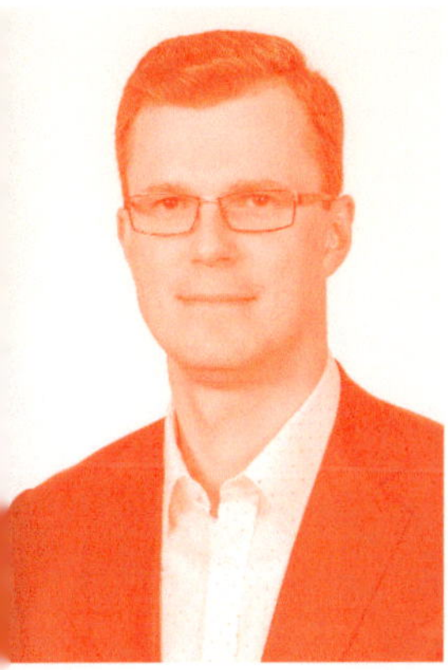
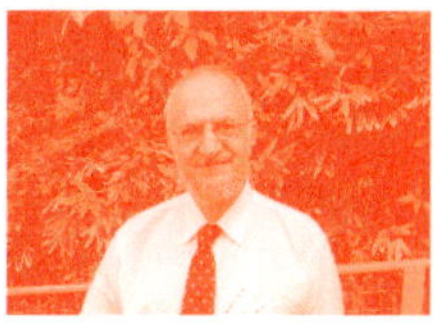
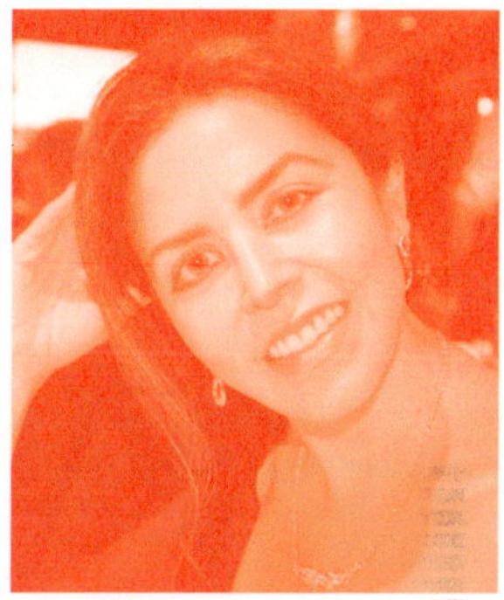

Supporting open minds since 2005

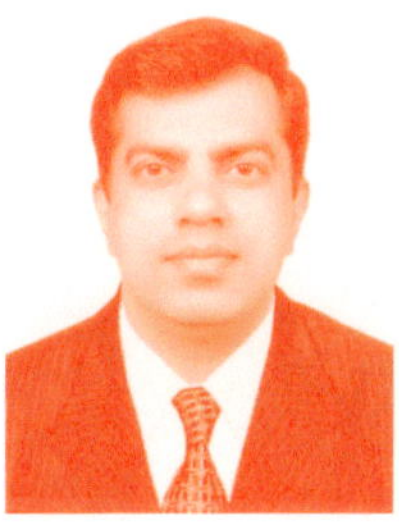
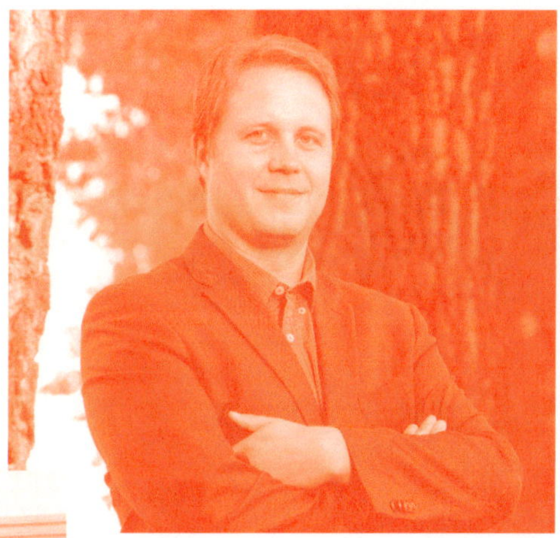
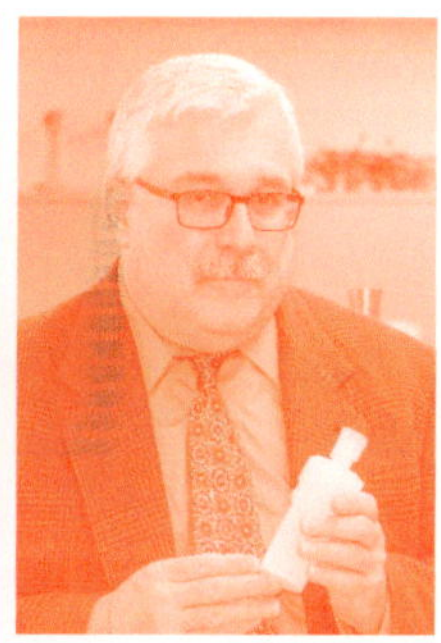
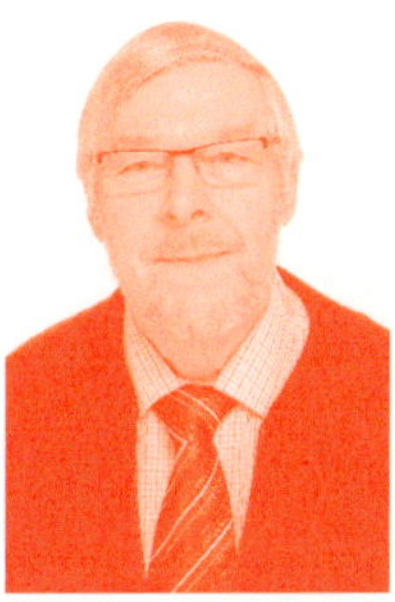
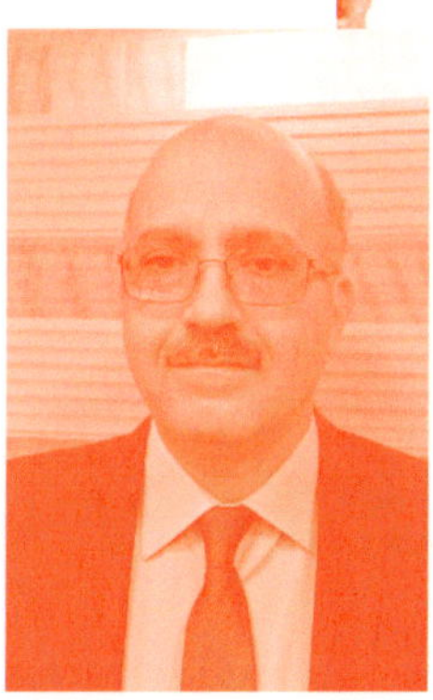
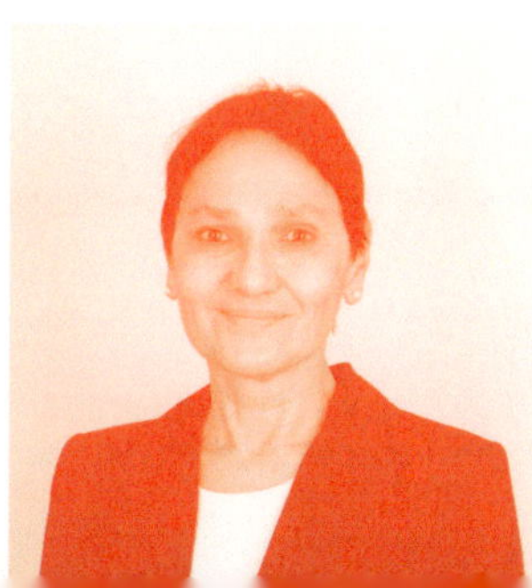
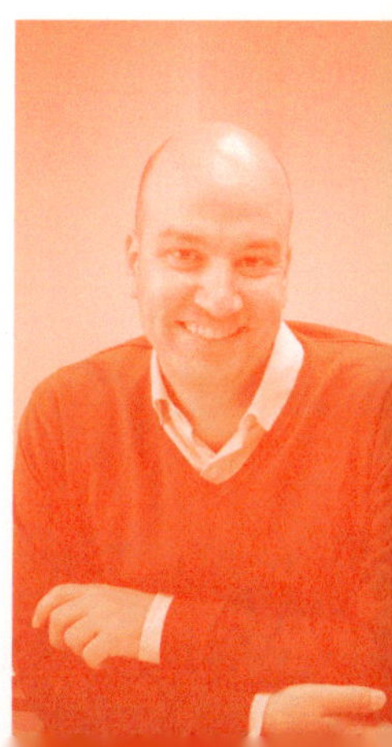

Muscular Dystrophy - Research Updates and Therapeutic Strategies
http://dx.doi.org/10.5772/intechopen.87261
Edited by Gisela Gaina

Contributors
Yuko Miyagoe-Suzuki, Ahmed Elhussieny, Kenichiro Nogami, Fusako Sakai-Takemura, Yusuke Maruyama, Abdelraouf Omar Abdelbakey, Wael Abou El-kheir, Shin'ichi Takeda, Jonathan Dando, Maximilian Lebmeier, Fleur Chandler, Josie Godfrey, Ahmed Osman, Nahla Mousa, Nagia Fahmy, Ahmed Abdellatif, Waheed Zahra, Mariia Sokolova, Ekaterina Valentinovna Lopatina, Amelia Aranega, Diego Franco, Estefania Lozano-Velasco, Lara Rodriguez-Outeiriño, Francisco Hernandez-Torres, Lidia María Matías Valiente, Robin Warner

First published in London, United Kingdom, 2021 by IntechOpen
IntechOpen is the global imprint of INTECHOPEN LIMITED, registered in England and Wales, registration number: 11086078, 5 Princes Gate Court, London, SW7 2QJ, United Kingdom
Printed in Croatia

British Library Cataloguing-in-Publication Data
A catalogue record for this book is available from the British Library

Additional hard and PDF copies can be obtained from orders@intechopen.com

Muscular Dystrophy - Research Updates and Therapeutic Strategies
Edited by Gisela Gaina
p. cm.
Print ISBN 978-1-83968-474-6
Online ISBN 978-1-83968-475-3
eBook (PDF) ISBN 978-1-83968-476-0

For EU product safety concerns:
IN TECH d.o.o., Prolaz Marije Krucifikse Kozulić 3, 51000 Rijeka, Croatia, info@intechopen.com or visit our website at intechopen.com.

Meet the editor

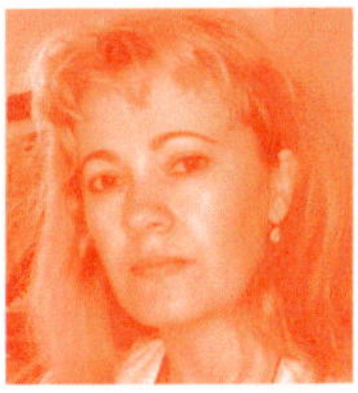

Florina Gisela Gaina, PhD, currently works at "Victor Babes" National Institute of Pathology, Bucharest, Romania. She received her PhD in Biology from the University of Bucharest, Romania, in 2009 with a thesis project based on the study of the proteins involved in muscular dystrophies. She is a research scientist working in the field of skeletal muscle. The primary focus of her research activities is on skeletal muscle regeneration. She has been involved in a number of research projects funded by regional, national, and international public agencies. She is an author and/or co-author of more than twenty scientific papers and conference abstracts and three book chapters.

Contents

Preface

Muscular dystrophies are a group of genetic disorders characterized by progressive weakness and loss of muscle mass. Although more than 30 years have passed since the discovery of the first protein involved in a type of muscular dystrophy, there is still no cure for these conditions. In the last decades, with the improvement of existing molecular biology techniques and the development of new approaches, many efforts have been made to accelerate the disease diagnostic process, to better understand the molecular defects and mechanisms underlying the molecular pathogenesis involved in dystrophy conditions.

Consequently, the development of different effective therapeutic strategies that slow down the course of the disease and improve patient quality of life and mortality continues to be a priority for researchers.

This book provides a comprehensive overview of the recent advances in the area of muscle diseases covering clinical manifestations, current diagnostic and therapeutic strategies, clinical trials, and their specific issues. In addition, this book updates the knowledge on mesenchymal stem/progenitor cells and miRNA, and discusses their therapeutic potential in regenerative medicine in a clear and concise manner.

We are very pleased to have had the opportunity to write this book on muscular dystrophy for IntechOpen, and we hope that this book will offer inspiration for young and experienced researchers to answer the many questions muscle pathology raises.

I would like to thank Author Service Manager Romina Rovan for her patience and valuable advice throughout the preparation of this book.

Florina Gisela Gaina
Victor Babes National Institute of Pathology,
Bucharest, Romania

Chapter 1

Duchenne Muscular Dystrophy (DMD) Treatment: Past and Present Perspectives

Nahla O. Mousa, Ahmed Osman, Nagia Fahmy, Ahmed Abdellatif and Waheed K. Zahra

Abstract

Duchenne muscular dystrophy (DMD) is one of the fatal X-linked disorders that are characterized by progressive muscle weakness and occur due to mutation in the largest human gene known as the DMD gene which encodes dystrophin protein that is mandatory for keeping the muscles structurally and functionally intact. The disease always affects boys (1 from every ~5000), and in some cases the female carriers are symptomatic. The disease usually leads to impairment in cardiac and pulmonary functions leading to the death of the patients in very young ages. Understanding DMD through precise molecular diagnosis will aid in determining the suitable therapeutic approach for the cases like designing exon-skipping antisense oligonucleotides (AOs) or stem cell-based therapies in conjunction with gene editing techniques (CRISPR/Cas9). Such therapies can correct the genetic defect in the DMD gene and ameliorate the symptoms. In this chapter, we will illustrate the past and current strategies for DMD disease treatment.

Keywords: DMD, exon skipping, CRISPR, cardiosphere, utrophin

1. Introduction

Duchenne muscular dystrophy (DMD) is a fatal X-linked disorder characterized by skeletal muscle wasting that is resulted from mutations in the dystrophin gene [1]. The disease occurs at a frequency of about 1 in ~5000 newborn males, making it the most common severe neuromuscular disease in humans. Dystrophin is present in normal individuals from fetal life onwards in all skeletal, cardiac, and smooth muscles; the absence of dystrophin protein causes muscle weakness and protein degradation and ultimately causes cell death. Death usually occurs in the third decade of life as the result of respiratory or heart failure [2]. The precise diagnosis for DMD should contain a combination of genetic testing after muscle biopsy and clinical observation of muscle strength and function.

The main current medication so far is corticosteroids, which have been shown to increase muscle strength in many studies. Genetic therapy using mini-/micro-dystrophin vectors, suppression of premature termination codon, exon-skipping antisense oligonucleotides (AOs) which bind with RNA and exclude specific sites of RNA splicing producing a dystrophin that is smaller but functional, and such new emerging drugs are the pass to the new era towards DMD treatment. In the next section, we will review all available FDA-approved treatments and recent research trials aiming at ameliorating DMD symptoms.

2. Methods for treatment

2.1 Corticosteroids

Corticosteroids were the first line of treatment for DMD; it was first used by Drachman et al. in 1974 [3] when they had promising positive results in their study after using prednisone (anti-inflammatory glucocorticosteroid). Since then, many studies were carried out to test the therapeutic effect of such treatment since it was found to improve muscle performance.

Deflazacart (DFZ), an oxazolidine derivative of prednisone, was used by an Italian group [4] and other groups [5–7], and the drug demonstrated efficiency in disease treatment and preserved lung function. The exact mechanism of DFZ is not yet known; however, it might regulate some signaling cascades. It was found to activate calcineurin/NF-AT pathway [8]. Also, DFZ may act by decreasing necrosis and muscle inflammation and reducing the degree of muscle degeneration. It can also act through modulating dystrophin expression and inducing the myogenesis in addition to having positive effects on muscular tissue mass [9].

Despite the advantages of using steroids, they also had side effects like gaining weight, affecting bone mineral density, which leads to vertebral fractures and behavioral changes. Furthermore, high dosages are required to reach the target effect and to be active at the site inflammation. Also, the drug can be accumulated in other nontargeted areas [10, 11].

In one of their studies, Luhder et al. [12] tried to improve the therapeutic effect of the steroids through developing an 80 nm PEGylated nano-liposome that is conjugated with the steroid prodrug “methylprednisolone hemisuccinate.” The results of their study showed that such structure was selectively targeting the diaphragm in vivo (using mdx mouse model) when administered intravenously and the treatment reduced the infiltration with macrophages and serum levels of transforming growth factor beta. Most importantly, the study showed that long-term use of this formulation leads to enhanced mobility and increased muscle strength.

2.2 Exon skipping

Exon skipping is considered as one of the mutation-based treatments for Duchenne muscular dystrophy [13]. In DMD, some deletions in specific exons lead to the disruption of the reading frame of the dystrophin protein, and consequently such deletions lead to the production of truncated product missing a huge part of the protein (usually missing the rod domain and C-terminal domain).

However, sometimes, deleting additional exons may restore the reading frame and lead to the production of dystrophin protein missing only a portion of the central rod domain while the C-terminal domain remains intact, and hence the protein product in this case is lacking specific regions, but it is semi-functional and can induce Becker-like symptoms instead of the complete loss of the muscular function [14].

The main idea of exon skipping is using the “antisense oligonucleotide” molecules to induce the skipping of a specific exon (other than the already mutated one) and prevent it from being translated to restore the reading frame. As an example, patients with exon 45 deletion could be treated through the skipping of an additional exon 44. Eteplirsen (Exondys51™) based on phosphorodiamidite morpholino oligomer (PMD) is an FDA-approved antisense treatment to skip exon 51 for patients with mutation ▲49–50 [15]. Also, drisapersen (based on 2′-O-methyl phosphorothioate; 2′-OMePS-modified AOs) is one of the AOs that are designed to treat DMD patients with mutations that can be ameliorated by exon 51 skipping; however it was not approved by the FDA [16, 17].

Various modifications can take place to the sugar of the oligonucleotide or to the backbone of the oligo. This could include phosphorodiamidate morpholino, locked nucleic acid (LNA), or peptide-conjugated oligo. Regarding the morpholinos, the oligonucleotide backbone is replaced with the morpholino backbone which makes the oligonucleotide nontoxic and has high affinity to RNA molecules. The locked nucleic acids are oligonucleotides that have a modified ribose sugar where the 2′ oxygen is connected with the 4′ carbon atom which creates a locked ribose ring. Also, the LNAs are nontoxic with superior affinity to complementary targeted RNA sequences [18].

The main problem in developing such treatments based on the skipping is that it will only fit a small group of patients (a mutation-specific AO should be developed for each group of patients and will not be suitable for other patients); also some patients have deletions in critical parts of the protein, and hence skipping of other exons will not have a therapeutic impact (**Table 1**).

2.3 Induced pluripotent stem cells along with genome editing technique

The sole cause of DMD is the presence of mutation that adversely affects the DMD gene. So, in order to permanently fix such mutations and treat this condition, patients could be provided with muscle cells harboring the normal copy of DMD gene. Since it is hard to get mature muscle fibers from a normal individual to be used as a source of healthy muscle cells with normal DMD gene, also the availability of such source of cells will not guarantee the process of grafting in the patient's muscles since it could be subjected to rejection by the body and can initiate an aggressive immune response. Cell reprogramming and genome editing techniques efficiently aid in solving this puzzling dilemma [25]. The process of cell reprogramming paved the road towards developing normal muscle fibers by starting with patient-specialized adult cells followed by inducing the production of induced pluripotent stem cells (iPSCs) (using the Nobel prize-winning technology of reprogramming using specific transcription factors like Oct4, Sox2, Klf4, and L-Myc) [26]. Also, some microRNAs have the potential to reprogram the adult cells efficiently (like miR-302b, miR-372) [27].

After the reprogramming and the production of stem cells, gene editing technologies should be used to correct the mutation of the gene. CRISPR/Cas 9 is now a leading technology that is presently considered as an avenue for DMD treatment; the RNA-guided DNA endonuclease system allows the correction of the DMD segment which is essential for dystrophin restoration [28, 29].

In order to conduct a gene editing experiment with CRISPR/Cas9 system, two important elements should be provided: guide RNA (gRNA) specific for the target gene and Cas9 nuclease (Sp. Cas9 (from *Streptococcus pyogenes*; 4.10 kb) or Sp. Cas9 (*Staphylococcus aureus*; 3.16 kb)) or Cj. Cas9 (*Campylobacter jejuni*; 2.95 kb) that can cleave DNA strands where the guide RNA is bound and in the presence of three- to five-nucleotide proto-spacer adjacent motif (PAM) sequence to be digested. Upon the binding of the gRNA, Cas9 can induce a double-strand break which is then repaired by the cell through the nonhomologous end joining, and this will initiate a repair mechanism in which nucleotides will be added or deleted at the cleaved site which can consequently restore the reading frame of the DMD gene to the normal

Chemistry	Route of administration	The used model	Treatment strategy	Treatment effects	Reference
Phosphorodiamidate morpholino oligomers (Ex6A, Ex6B, Ex8A, and Ex8G)	Intravenous	Neonatal CXMDJ	Exon 6–9 skipping	Dystrophin restoration across skeletal muscles (14% of healthy levels) Reduction of fibrosis and/or necrosis area	[19]
Phosphorodiamidate morpholino oligomer (NS-065/NCNP-01)	Endo-Porter reagent	Fibroblasts from patients with DMD involving deletion of exons 45–52 or exons 48–52 and injected with MYOD for myotube differentiation	Exon 53 skipping	Restored dystrophin protein levels in the cells	[20]
Phosphorodiamidate morpholino oligomer	Intramuscular and intravenous	mdx52 mouse model	Exon 51 skipping	Only the protocol was mentioned	[21]
Phosphorodiamidate morpholino oligomer (NS-065/NCNP-01)	Intravenous	Patients with DMD	Exon 53 skipping	Increased dystrophin/spectrin ratio in 7 of 10 patients in TA muscle biopsies	[22]
Pip6a-PMO; PMOME23, sequence GGCCAAACCTCGGCTT-ACCTGAAAT	Intravenous	Cmah-/-mdx mice	Exon 23 skipping	Dystrophin restoration in the heart Reduction in myocardial fibrosis Reducing maximum pressure and arterial elastance	[23]
Inhibitor of CDC2-like kinase 1 (named TG693)	Oral Lipofectamine reagent	Male Jcl:TCR mice Patient-derived myotubes	Exon 31 skipping	It induces exon skipping and restored dystrophin expression in patient-derived cells. And it modulated splicing in mouse skeletal muscle	[24]
Morpholino AOs targeting DMD exon 51	Endo-Porter transfection Intramuscular	Immortalized DMD muscle cells hDMD/Dmd null mice	Exon 51 skipping	The rescue of dystrophin protein expression	[25]

Table 1.
Studies conducted on treatment of DMD using exon skipping (during 2017–2019).

ORF. In some cases, single (or several) gRNA molecule could be designed to target splicing sites which can lead to the skipping of specific exon leading to the production of functional proteins. Additionally, base editing mediated by CRISPR/Cas9 could be obtained through Cas9 enzymes lacking the nuclease activity, so it can induce only a single-strand break. Such enzymes can catalyze base editing (A:T to G:C) through having a cytidine deaminase activity [30].

Ousterout et al. in their study used another editing protocol (zinc finger nuclease) to delete exon 51 from the transcript from patient-derived myoblasts [31]. Also, Young et al. carried out CRISPR/Cas9 experiment utilizing a single pair of guide RNAs to delete exons 45–55 in iPSC, and such deletion leads to the expression of stable dystrophin protein with improved membrane stability in derived skeletal myotubes and cardiomyocytes [32]. Another study by Duchene et al. utilized a single guide RNA to produce a hybrid exon which led to the production of functional dystrophin protein with completely normal structure [33]. The main advantage of this reprogramming protocol is that it allows performing an autologous grafting of the muscle cells to patients.

For the expression of the specific gRNA molecules inside the muscle cells, adeno-associated virus (AAV) vectors will be used. Sometimes, the expression of the gRNAs can lead to off-target effect due to the incorrect binding with another similar DNA sequence inside the host cell. In order to avoid this damaging effect, AAV vectors expressing multiple gRNA molecules could be used.

After the completion of the gene editing process, the edited cells would be treated with myogenic factors to convert the edited stem cells again to myoblasts for the myogenic differentiation (**Table 2**).

2.4 Gene therapy

Gene therapy is one of the most appealing techniques that are used to deliver a normal copy of the DMD gene to express the fully functional dystrophin protein. This method implies injecting the patients with plasmids carrying normal dystrophin cDNA (~12 kb).

In 2002, the first phase 1 trial of DMD gene therapy took place using full-length dystrophin [52]. After that, adeno-associated viral vectors carrying mini forms of dystrophin cDNA were used for gene therapy, and this was better regarding the packaging size of the plasmids, and it is much easier to transfer/deliver mini forms of DMD gene [53, 54].

However, such therapeutic approach faced another problem which is the distribution of the plasmids across all affected muscular tissue that is spreading all over the body, and that is why microdystrophin plasmids and systemic AAV delivery were developed and improved to solve such problem. Evidence from many trials using animal models revealed that gene therapy can lead to long-term expression of functional protein [55–57].

In 2017, Le Guiner et al. studied the effect of the delivery of rAAV2/8 vector expressing a canine microdystrophin (cMD1) in golden retriever muscular dystrophy (GRMD) dogs in the absence of immunosuppression. Such treatment affected the deterioration of the muscular activity, and the gene expression was maintained over a long period [56]. Recently in 2020, Genthon and Sarepta contracted Yposkesi for manufacturing the AAV microdystrophin vector on a large scale.

2.5 Dystrophin-expressing chimeric cells

As previously mentioned, the absence of dystrophin is the main cause of DMD disease and the aggressive symptoms including muscle weakness and degeneration

Plasmids (source of Cas9 and guide RNAs)	Route of administration	The used model	Treatment strategy	Reference
Adeno-associated viral vectors of serotype 9 carrying an intein-split Cas9 A pair of guide RNAs targeting sequences flanking exon 51 (AAV9-Cas9-gE51)	Intramuscular injection	DMDΔ52 pigs	Excision of exon 51	[34]
SaCas9 expression plasmid Two gRNA expression cassettes driven by the human U6 pol. III promoter (AAV8 and AAV9)	Locally in the TA muscles	C57BL/10ScSn-Dmdmdx/J	Excision of exon 23	[35]
pSpCas9 expression plasmid AAV TRISPR-sgRNA-CK8e-GFP plasmid contained three sgRNAs driven by the U6, H1, or 7SK promoter and green florescent protein (GFP) driven by the CK8e regulatory cassette	Transfection reagent Locally in the TA muscles	Human DMD-derived iPSCs ▲Exon 44 DMD mice	Excision of exons 43 and 45	[36]
Streptococcus pyogenes Cas9 Single guide RNA (sgRNA-51) (AAV9-Cas9 and AAV9-sgRNA-51)	Locally in the cranial tibialis muscles	▲Exon 50 canine model	Excision of exon 51	[37]
spCas9 and crDMDint2.1 and int2.6 gRNAs	Transfection reagent (linear polyethylenimine derivative)	Immortalized myoblasts from DMD patient	Excision of duplicated exon 2	[38]
Lenti-V2-Ugi-nCas9-AIDx or Lenti-V2-AIDx-nSaCas9 (KKH)-Ugi (2.5 μg) and pCDNA3 Ugi	Transfection reagent (lipid-based)	▲51-iPSCs of a male DMD patient	Excision of exon 50	[39]
CRISPR-Cas9 variant (D10A Cas9 nickase (nCas9) or catalytically deficient D10A/H840A Cas9 (dCas9) from *S. pyogenes*) and a deaminase protein from various sources sgRNA (gX20) under the control of the U6 promoter (pAAV-ITR-ABE-NT-sgRNA)	Micromanipulator	Mouse zygote from DMD knockout mouse	Base editing of exon 20	[40]
Plasmids containing regulatory cassettes for expression of Cas9 or gRNAs flanked by AAV serotype 2 inverted terminal repeats (ITRs)	Electroporation Intramuscular	Fibroblasts isolated from male mdx4cv mice Male mdx4cv mice	Excision of exons 52 and 53	[41]

Plasmids (source of Cas9 and guide RNAs)	Route of administration	The used model	Treatment strategy	Reference
pX601-AAV CMV::NLS-SaCas9-NLS-3xHA-bGHpA;U6::BsaI-sgRNA (PX601)	Transfection reagent (lipid-based)	Myoblasts	Excision of exons 47 and 48	[33]
		DMD iPSC	Excision of exons 44–55	[32]
The gRNA cassettes gI43, gI52, gI53, and gI54.2 (targeting different introns) controlled by human U6 RNA polymerase III promoter Plasmids AU53_pAd Shu.gI52.gI53.PGK.Cas9.SV40pA, plasmids pLV.gI52 and pLV.gI53	Transduction (by gelatin)	DMD myoblasts Δ48–50 and Δ45–52	Excision of exon 53	[42]
pAAV-ITR-CjCas9-sgRNA, pAAV2/9 encoding for AAV2rep and AAV9cap, and helper plasmid	Intramuscular in the TA muscle	Knockout mice	Excision of exon 23	[43]
pSpCas9(BB)-2A-GFP (PX458)	Transfection reagent	DMD hiPSCs, hiPSC-derived cardiac muscle cells	Excision of exon 51, introns 47, 50, 54	[44]
pSpCas9(BB)-2A-GFP (PX458)	Intramuscular in the TA muscle	Mice ▲50	Excision of exon 51	[45]
Purified Cas9 protein and in vitro transcribed gRNA	Gold nanoparticles	Primary myoblasts C57BL/10ScSn-Dmdmdx/J (mdx) mice	Excision of exon 23	[46]
pSpCas9(BB)-2A-GFP (PX458)	Nucleofection	Induced pluripotent stem cells (iPSCs)	Deleting exons 3–9, 6–9, or 7–11	[47]
Nuclease-expressing plasmids (TALENs, left and right; CRISPR, Cas9 and sgRNA)	Electroporation	DMD fibroblasts were derived from a DMD patient lacking exon 44	Excision of exon 45	[48]
Cas9 mixed with 44C1, 44C2, 45C2, and 45C3 gRNAs produced via in vitro transcription	Electroporation	hDMD (Tg(DMD)72Thoen/J, 018900), C57BL/10 mdx (001801), and mdxD2 (D1.B10-Dmdmdx/J, 013141)	Excision of exons 45–55	[49]

Plasmids (source of Cas9 and guide RNAs)	Route of administration	The used model	Treatment strategy	Reference
AdV-Cas9-RFP AdG-gRNA-Donor	Transfection reagent (lipid based)	Skeletal muscle cell culture derived from C57BL/10ScSn-Dmd mdx/J	Excision of exon 23	[50]
Cpf1 gRNAs targeting the human DMD or the mouse Dmd locus (subcloned into pLbCpf1-2A-GFP and pAsCpf1-2A-GFP)	Nucleofection	DMD iPSC cells	Excision of exon 51	[51]

Table 2.
Studies conducted on treatment of DMD using gene editing techniques (CRISPR/Cas9) (during 2017–2020).

of muscle fibers. Such defect in the DMD gene can be edited using gene editing technology; however such technology can lead to off-target mutations which consequently can have damaging effects, and that is why more therapies had to be developed to address the disadvantages of such techniques.

Chimeric cell therapy is an alternative therapeutic approach that is usually done through the fusion of normal myoblasts and dystrophin-deficient myoblasts using polyethylene glycol (PEG). The success of this process could be tested using immunophenotyping (flow cytometry) and dystrophin immunostaining. This fusion will be followed by transplantation of chimeric cells in the defected muscle. The chimeric cells always show behavior like the donor cells regarding dystrophin expression and myogenic differentiation, and this dramatically improves the muscle function after being transplanted [58].

2.6 Cardiosphere-derived cells (CDCs)

Cardiosphere-derived cells are a type of cells that are retrieved from cardiac explants that can be cultured in vitro. Such cells have anti-inflammatory, antioxidant, and antibiotic activities. Several studies tested the ability of CDCs to alter the pathophysiology of DMD after the injection of these cells directly into the cardiac muscle.

Recently it was found that using CDCs greatly enhanced the phenotypic status of cardiac and skeletal muscles. The therapeutic effects of CDCs are usually attributed to the secretion of specific exosomes carrying specific genetic material to distal cells to exert its biological effect. Such CDCs along with their secreted exosomes can be injected intravenously, and it was found that they can greatly enhance the skeletal and cardiac muscle functions and boost the muscle generation process [59, 60].

2.7 Stop codon read-through therapy

In some of the mutations affecting the DMD gene, a premature stop codon is produced that can significantly disturb the reading frame and gives a truncated abnormal protein that cannot maintain the structural and functional properties of the muscle fibers.

A class of antibiotics called aminoglycosides was found to bind to rRNA at their decoding sites, preventing the stop codons from being read by binding to the A site (acceptor site) in the ribosomes and forcing the cell to prevent reading the stop codon, hence leading to the production of fully functional proteins.

PTC124 (ataluren; trade name, Translarna™) is one of the drugs with the read-through properties that are used for the treatment of DMD. Clinical trials showed that this drug when administered orally induced the expression of the dystrophin protein.

However, this treatment can only be used in ~15% of the cases who have a stop signal resulted from point mutation in the DMD gene. Also, it must be administered in increasing doses; beside it has many side effects such as renal toxicity. That is why there is a need to develop other alternatives with other structures to be safer with chronic usage.

2.8 Utrophin modulation

Recently, DMD symptoms were found to be managed after the administration of utrophin protein expression enhancers (utrophin is a dystrophin homolog; 395 KDa in size) to DMD patients delays the need of wheelchair and efficiently substitutes non-functional dystrophin.

Like dystrophin, the utrophin is present in the sarcolemma in the first developmental stages, and then replacement with dystrophin took place during muscular maturation. However, utrophin was found to be present in the myotendinous junction in adults. Interestingly, the expression of utrophin becomes elevated as a normal repair mechanism to compensate the absence of functional dystrophin in regenerated muscles.

SMTC-1100 is one of the chemical molecules that showed a great potential to increase the expression of DMD transcript and protein as well. This drug can be administered orally, if it was found to be safe and well tolerated in volunteers. However further studies are still required to detect if high dosage of this drug is safe or not.

Recently, ASA or adenylo-succinic acid improved the status of the TA muscles in mdx mice after administration of this compound in the drinking water. This molecule regulated the expression of the utrophin protein and hence greatly reduced the damaged area [61].

Another study group designed AAV vector carrying mini forms of the utrophin protein (μUtro). Their results showed that expression of this functional copy of utrophin protein (dystrophin analogue) after administration of the utrophin vector in DMD animal models completely reduced the muscle necrosis and regeneration [62].

3. Conclusion

Many medications have been used for DMD treatment and for preventing further deterioration of the cases. Corticosteroids were the first line of effective therapy of DMD; however, it does not modify the genetic mutations of the gene and does not affect the expression levels of dystrophin protein. Consequently, other treatments were developed including read-through stop codon, gene therapies, and exon skipping AOs which modulate and upregulate the levels of functional dystrophin transcript and protein in the muscles. Genome editing technology is also a powerful tool that can treat DMD permanently through the correction of the mutated sequence of DMD gene through the administration of sequence-specific guide RNA strands to bind selectively in the sequence to be edited. Also upregulating utrophin can help in the management of the cases. In addition, dystrophin-expressing chimeric cells and cardiosphere-derived cells are two emerging techniques that have the potential to treat DMD. Other medications will be developed to treat all DMD patients with different mutations with minimum side effects and maximum improvement in the status of the muscular system.

Author details

Nahla O. Mousa[1,2], Ahmed Osman[1,3]*, Nagia Fahmy[4], Ahmed Abdellatif[5] and Waheed K. Zahra[6,7]

1 Biotechnology Department, Basic and Applied Sciences Institute, Egypt-Japan University of Science and Technology, Borg El Arab, Egypt

2 Biotechnology Department, Faculty of Science, Cairo University, Giza, Egypt

3 Biochemistry Department, Faculty of Science, Ain Shams University, Cairo, Egypt

4 Neuromuscular Unit, Faculty of Medicine, Neuropsychiatry Department, Ain Shams University, Cairo, Egypt

5 Biology Department, School of Sciences and Engineering, The American University in Cairo, Cairo, Egypt

6 Mathematics Department, Basic and Applied Sciences Institute, Egypt-Japan University of Science and Technology, Borg El Arab, Egypt

7 Mathematics Department, Faculty of Engineering, Tanta University, Tanta, Egypt

*Address all correspondence to: ahmed.osman@ejust.edu.eg

References

[1] Hoffman EP, Brown RH Jr, Kunkel LM. Dystrophin: The protein product of the Duchenne muscular dystrophy locus. Cell. 1987;**51**(6):919-928

[2] Gao QQ, McNally EM. The dystrophin complex: Structure, function, and implications for therapy. Comprehensive Physiology. 2015;**5**(3):1223-1239

[3] Drachman DB, Toyka KV, Myer E. Prednisone in Duchenne muscular dystrophy. Lancet. 1974;**2**(7894):1409-1412

[4] Angelini C, Pegoraro E, Turella E, Intino MT, Pini A, Costa C. Deflazacort in Duchenne dystrophy: Study of long-term effect. Muscle & Nerve. 1994;**17**(4):386-391

[5] Bonifati MD, Ruzza G, Bonometto P, Berardinelli A, Gorni K, Orcesi S, et al. A multicenter, double-blind, randomized trial of deflazacort versus prednisone in Duchenne muscular dystrophy. Muscle & Nerve. 2000;**23**(9):1344-1347

[6] Biggar WD, Harris VA, Eliasoph L, Alman B. Long-term benefits of deflazacort treatment for boys with Duchenne muscular dystrophy in their second decade. Neuromuscular Disorders. 2006;**16**(4):249-255

[7] Biggar WD, Politano L, Harris VA, Passamano L, Vajsar J, Alman B, et al. Deflazacort in Duchenne muscular dystrophy: A comparison of two different protocols. Neuromuscular Disorders. 2004;**14**(8-9):476-482

[8] St-Pierre SJ, Chakkalakal JV, Kolodziejczyk SM, Knudson JC, Jasmin BJ, Megeney LA. Glucocorticoid treatment alleviates dystrophic myofiber pathology by activation of the calcineurin/NF-AT pathway. The FASEB Journal. 2004;**18**(15):1937-1939

[9] Jensen L, Petersson SJ, Illum NO, Laugaard-Jacobsen HC, Thelle T, Jorgensen LH, et al. Muscular response to the first three months of deflazacort treatment in boys with Duchenne muscular dystrophy. Journal of Musculoskeletal & Neuronal Interactions. 2017;**17**(2):8-18

[10] McAdam LC, Mayo AL, Alman BA, Biggar WD. The Canadian experience with long-term deflazacort treatment in Duchenne muscular dystrophy. Acta Myologica. 2012;**31**(1):16-20

[11] Lippuner K, Casez JP, Horber FF, Jaeger P. Effects of deflazacort versus prednisone on bone mass, body composition, and lipid profile: A randomized, double blind study in kidney transplant patients. The Journal of Clinical Endocrinology and Metabolism. 1998;**83**(11):3795-3802

[12] Luhder F, Reichardt HM. Novel drug delivery systems tailored for improved administration of glucocorticoids. International Journal of Molecular Sciences. 2017;**18**(9):1836

[13] Echevarria L, Aupy P, Goyenvalle A. Exon-skipping advances for Duchenne muscular dystrophy. Human Molecular Genetics. 2018;**27**(R2):R163-RR72

[14] Aartsma-Rus A, Fokkema I, Verschuuren J, Ginjaar I, van Deutekom J, van Ommen GJ, et al. Theoretic applicability of antisense-mediated exon skipping for Duchenne muscular dystrophy mutations. Human Mutation. 2009;**30**(3):293-299

[15] Charleston JS, Schnell FJ, Dworzak J, Donoghue C, Lewis S, Chen L, et al. Eteplirsen treatment for Duchenne muscular dystrophy: Exon

skipping and dystrophin production. Neurology. 2018;**90**(24):e2146-e2e54

[16] Goemans N, Mercuri E, Belousova E, Komaki H, Dubrovsky A, McDonald CM, et al. A randomized placebo-controlled phase 3 trial of an antisense oligonucleotide, drisapersen, in Duchenne muscular dystrophy. Neuromuscular Disorders. 2018;**28**(1):4-15

[17] McDonald CM, Wong B, Flanigan KM, Wilson R, de Kimpe S, Lourbakos A, et al. Placebo-controlled phase 2 trial of drisapersen for Duchenne muscular dystrophy. Annals of Clinical Translational Neurology. 2018;**5**(8):913-926

[18] Aartsma-Rus A, Kaman WE, Bremmer-Bout M, Janson AA, den Dunnen JT, van Ommen GJ, et al. Comparative analysis of antisense oligonucleotide analogs for targeted DMD exon 46 skipping in muscle cells. Gene Therapy. 2004;**11**(18):1391-1398

[19] Lim KRQ, Echigoya Y, Nagata T, Kuraoka M, Kobayashi M, Aoki Y, et al. Efficacy of multi-exon skipping treatment in Duchenne muscular dystrophy dog model neonates. Molecular Therapy. 2019;**27**(1):76-86

[20] Watanabe N, Nagata T, Satou Y, Masuda S, Saito T, Kitagawa H, et al. NS-065/NCNP-01: An antisense oligonucleotide for potential treatment of exon 53 skipping in Duchenne muscular dystrophy. Molecular Therapy—Nucleic Acids. 2018;**13**:442-449

[21] Miyatake S, Mizobe Y, Takizawa H, Hara Y, Yokota T, Takeda S, et al. Exon skipping therapy using phosphorodiamidate morpholino oligomers in the mdx52 mouse model of Duchenne muscular dystrophy. Methods in Molecular Biology. 2018;**1687**:123-141

[22] Komaki H, Nagata T, Saito T, Masuda S, Takeshita E, Sasaki M, et al. Systemic administration of the antisense oligonucleotide NS-065/NCNP-01 for skipping of exon 53 in patients with Duchenne muscular dystrophy. Science Translational Medicine. 2018;**10**(437)

[23] Blain AM, Greally E, McClorey G, Manzano R, Betts CA, Godfrey C, et al. Peptide-conjugated phosphodiamidate oligomer-mediated exon skipping has benefits for cardiac function in mdx and Cmah-/-mdx mouse models of Duchenne muscular dystrophy. PLOS One. 2018;**13**(6):e0198897

[24] Sako Y, Ninomiya K, Okuno Y, Toyomoto M, Nishida A, Koike Y, et al. Development of an orally available inhibitor of CLK1 for skipping a mutated dystrophin exon in Duchenne muscular dystrophy. Scientific Reports. 2017;**7**:46126

[25] Echigoya Y, Lim KRQ, Trieu N, Bao B, Miskew Nichols B, Vila MC, et al. Quantitative antisense screening and optimization for exon 51 skipping in Duchenne muscular dystrophy. Molecular Therapy. 2017;**25**(11):2561-2572

[26] Danisovic L, Culenova M, Csobonyeiova M. Induced pluripotent stem cells for Duchenne muscular dystrophy modeling and therapy. Cell. 2018;**7**(12):253

[27] Miyoshi N, Ishii H, Nagano H, Haraguchi N, Dewi DL, Kano Y, et al. Reprogramming of mouse and human cells to pluripotency using mature microRNAs. Cell Stem Cell. 2011;**8**(6):633-638

[28] Duchene B, Iyombe-Engembe JP, Rousseau J, Tremblay JP, Ouellet DL. From gRNA identification to the restoration of dystrophin expression: A dystrophin gene correction strategy for Duchenne muscular dystrophy

mutations using the CRISPR-induced deletion method. Methods in Molecular Biology. 2018;**1687**:267-283

[29] Min YL, Bassel-Duby R, Olson EN. CRISPR correction of Duchenne muscular dystrophy. Annual Review of Medicine. 2019;**70**:239-255

[30] Adli M. The CRISPR tool kit for genome editing and beyond. Nature Communications. 2018;**9**(1):1911

[31] Ousterout DG, Kabadi AM, Thakore PI, Perez-Pinera P, Brown MT, Majoros WH, et al. Correction of dystrophin expression in cells from Duchenne muscular dystrophy patients through genomic excision of exon 51 by zinc finger nucleases. Molecular Therapy. 2015;**23**(3):523-532

[32] Young CS, Hicks MR, Ermolova NV, Nakano H, Jan M, Younesi S, et al. A single CRISPR-Cas9 deletion strategy that targets the majority of DMD patients restores dystrophin function in hiPSC-derived muscle cells. Cell Stem Cell. 2016;**18**(4):533-540

[33] Duchene BL, Cherif K, Iyombe-Engembe JP, Guyon A, Rousseau J, Ouellet DL, et al. CRISPR-induced deletion with SaCas9 restores dystrophin expression in dystrophic models in vitro and in vivo. Molecular Therapy. 2018;**26**(11):2604-2616

[34] Moretti A, Fonteyne L, Giesert F, Hoppmann P, Meier AB, Bozoglu T, et al. Somatic gene editing ameliorates skeletal and cardiac muscle failure in pig and human models of Duchenne muscular dystrophy. Nature Medicine. 2020;**26**(2):207-214

[35] Nelson CE, Wu Y, Gemberling MP, Oliver ML, Waller MA, Bohning JD, et al. Long-term evaluation of AAV-CRISPR genome editing for Duchenne muscular dystrophy. Nature Medicine. 2019;**25**(3):427-432

[36] Min YL, Li H, Rodriguez-Caycedo C, Mireault AA, Huang J, Shelton JM, et al. CRISPR-Cas9 corrects Duchenne muscular dystrophy exon 44 deletion mutations in mice and human cells. Science Advances. 2019;**5**(3):eaav4324

[37] Amoasii L, Hildyard JCW, Li H, Sanchez-Ortiz E, Mireault A, Caballero D, et al. Gene editing restores dystrophin expression in a canine model of Duchenne muscular dystrophy. Science. 2018;**362**(6410):86-91

[38] Lattanzi A, Duguez S, Moiani A, Izmiryan A, Barbon E, Martin S, et al. Correction of the exon 2 duplication in DMD myoblasts by a single CRISPR/Cas9 system. Molecular Therapy--Nucleic Acids. 2017;**7**:11-19

[39] Yuan J, Ma Y, Huang T, Chen Y, Peng Y, Li B, et al. Genetic modulation of RNA splicing with a CRISPR-guided cytidine deaminase. Molecular Cell. 2018;**72**(2):380-394.e7

[40] Ryu SM, Koo T, Kim K, Lim K, Baek G, Kim ST, et al. Adenine base editing in mouse embryos and an adult mouse model of Duchenne muscular dystrophy. Nature Biotechnology. 2018;**36**(6):536-539

[41] Bengtsson NE, Hall JK, Odom GL, Phelps MP, Andrus CR, Hawkins RD, et al. Muscle-specific CRISPR/Cas9 dystrophin gene editing ameliorates pathophysiology in a mouse model for Duchenne muscular dystrophy. Nature Communications. 2017;**8**:14454

[42] Maggio I, Liu J, Janssen JM, Chen X, Goncalves MA. Adenoviral vectors encoding CRISPR/Cas9 multiplexes rescue dystrophin synthesis in unselected populations of DMD muscle cells. Scientific Reports. 2016;**6**:37051

[43] Koo T, Lu-Nguyen NB, Malerba A, Kim E, Kim D, Cappellari O, et al.

Functional rescue of dystrophin deficiency in mice caused by frameshift mutations using *Campylobacter jejuni* Cas9. Molecular Therapy. 2018;**26**(6):1529-1538

[44] Long C, Li H, Tiburcy M, Rodriguez-Caycedo C, Kyrychenko V, Zhou H, et al. Correction of diverse muscular dystrophy mutations in human engineered heart muscle by single-site genome editing. Science Advances. 2018;**4**(1):eaap9004

[45] Amoasii L, Long C, Li H, Mireault AA, Shelton JM, Sanchez-Ortiz E, et al. Single-cut genome editing restores dystrophin expression in a new mouse model of muscular dystrophy. Science Translational Medicine. 2017;**9**(418):eaan8081

[46] Lee K, Conboy M, Park HM, Jiang F, Kim HJ, Dewitt MA, et al. Nanoparticle delivery of Cas9 ribonucleoprotein and donor DNA in vivo induces homology-directed DNA repair. Nature Biomedical Engineering. 2017;**1**:889-901

[47] Kyrychenko V, Kyrychenko S, Tiburcy M, Shelton JM, Long C, Schneider JW, et al. Functional correction of dystrophin actin binding domain mutations by genome editing. JCI Insight. 2017;**2**(18):e95918

[48] Li HL, Fujimoto N, Sasakawa N, Shirai S, Ohkame T, Sakuma T, et al. Precise correction of the dystrophin gene in Duchenne muscular dystrophy patient induced pluripotent stem cells by TALEN and CRISPR-Cas9. Stem Cell Reports. 2015;**4**(1):143-154

[49] Young CS, Mokhonova E, Quinonez M, Pyle AD, Spencer MJ. Creation of a novel humanized dystrophic mouse model of Duchenne muscular dystrophy and application of a CRISPR/Cas9 gene editing therapy. Journal of Neuromuscular Diseases. 2017;**4**(2):139-145

[50] Zhu P, Wu F, Mosenson J, Zhang H, He TC, Wu WS. CRISPR/Cas9-mediated genome editing corrects dystrophin mutation in skeletal muscle stem cells in a mouse model of muscle dystrophy. Molecular Therapy--Nucleic Acids. 2017;7:31-41

[51] Zhang Y, Long C, Li H, McAnally JR, Baskin KK, Shelton JM, et al. CRISPR-Cpf1 correction of muscular dystrophy mutations in human cardiomyocytes and mice. Science Advances. 2017;**3**(4):e1602814

[52] DelloRusso C, Scott JM, Hartigan-O'Connor D, Salvatori G, Barjot C, Robinson AS, et al. Functional correction of adult mdx mouse muscle using gutted adenoviral vectors expressing full-length dystrophin. Proceedings of the National Academy of Sciences of the United States of America. 2002;**99**(20):12979-12984

[53] Sakamoto M, Yuasa K, Yoshimura M, Yokota T, Ikemoto T, Suzuki M, et al. Micro-dystrophin cDNA ameliorates dystrophic phenotypes when introduced into mdx mice as a transgene. Biochemical and Biophysical Research Communications. 2002;**293**(4):1265-1272

[54] Harper SQ, Hauser MA, DelloRusso C, Duan D, Crawford RW, Phelps SF, et al. Modular flexibility of dystrophin: Implications for gene therapy of Duchenne muscular dystrophy. Nature Medicine. 2002;**8**(3):253-261

[55] Koo T, Okada T, Athanasopoulos T, Foster H, Takeda S, Dickson G. Long-term functional adeno-associated virus-microdystrophin expression in the dystrophic CXMDj dog. The Journal of Gene Medicine. 2011;**13**(9):497-506

[56] Le Guiner C, Servais L, Montus M, Larcher T, Fraysse B, Moullec S, et al. Long-term microdystrophin gene

therapy is effective in a canine model of Duchenne muscular dystrophy. Nature Communications. 2017;**8**:16105

[57] Yoshimura M, Sakamoto M, Ikemoto M, Mochizuki Y, Yuasa K, Miyagoe-Suzuki Y, et al. AAV vector-mediated microdystrophin expression in a relatively small percentage of mdx myofibers improved the mdx phenotype. Molecular Therapy. 2004;**10**(5):821-828

[58] Siemionow M, Cwykiel J, Heydemann A, Garcia-Martinez J, Siemionow K, Szilagyi E. Creation of dystrophin expressing chimeric cells of myoblast origin as a novel stem cell based therapy for Duchenne muscular dystrophy. Stem Cell Reviews and Reports. 2018;**14**(2):189-199

[59] Rogers RG, Fournier M, Sanchez L, Ibrahim AG, Aminzadeh MA, Lewis MI, et al. Disease-modifying bioactivity of intravenous cardiosphere-derived cells and exosomes in mdx mice. JCI Insight. 2019;**4**(7):e125754

[60] Aminzadeh MA, Rogers RG, Fournier M, Tobin RE, Guan X, Childers MK, et al. Exosome-mediated benefits of cell therapy in mouse and human models of Duchenne muscular dystrophy. Stem Cell Reports. 2018;**10**(3):942-955

[61] Timpani CA, Goodman CA, Stathis CG, White JD, Mamchaoui K, Butler-Browne G, et al. Adenylosuccinic acid therapy ameliorates murine Duchenne muscular dystrophy. Scientific Reports. 2020;**10**(1):1125

[62] Song Y, Morales L, Malik AS, Mead AF, Greer CD, Mitchell MA, et al. Non-immunogenic utrophin gene therapy for the treatment of muscular dystrophy animal models. Nature Medicine. 2019;**25**(10):1505-1511

Chapter 2

Facioscapulohumeral Muscular Dystrophy: Genetics and Trials

Robin Warner

Abstract

A complex combination of molecular pathways and cell interactions causes facioscapulohumeral muscular dystrophy (FSHD). Several new therapies pose a promising solution to this disease with no cure. This chapter aims to explain the genetics of facioscapulohumeral muscular dystrophy, and review the current clinical trials for the treatment of FSHD.

Keywords: facioscapulohumeral muscular dystrophy, antisense oligonucleotide, decoy nucleic acid, novel therapies, genetics, trials

1. Introduction

1.1 Epidemiology

Facioscapulohumeral muscular dystrophy (FSHD) is one of the most common muscular dystrophies. Worldwide, its prevalence is up to 6.8 in 100,000 and in the United States, it is about 1 in 20,000. It affects men more than women because estrogens counteract the differentiation impairment of FSHD myoblasts without affecting cell proliferation or survival. Estrogen effects are mediated by estrogen receptor β (ERβ), which reduces chromatin occupancy and transcriptional activity of double homeobox 4 (DUX4) [1].

1.2 History

Facioscapulohumeral muscular dystrophy was first described by two French physicians, Louis Landouzy and Joseph Jules Dejerine, in the late 1800s [2]. Their description was based on a family that they had monitored for 11 years. In 1950, Tyler and Stephens described a family from Utah that included 1249 people spanning six generations. All were descendants of an affected individual who had migrated to Utah in 1840. Their findings confirmed the autosomal dominant inheritance pattern of FSHD. Clinical criteria were established by an international consortium in 1991. These criteria were as follows: onset of the disease in the facial or shoulder girdle muscles and sparing of the extraocular, pharyngeal, and lingual muscles and the myocardium, facial muscle weakness in more than 50% of affected family members, autosomal dominant inheritance in familial cases and evidence of myopathic disease from electromyography and muscle biopsy in at least one affected member, without biopsy features specific for alternative diagnoses.

2. Genetics

Facioscapulohumeral muscular dystrophy is caused by the inappropriate expression of an early embryonic transcriptional activator, DUX4, in adult muscle, leading to cell death [3, 4]. The disease is autosomal dominant, although up to one-third of cases involve de novo mutations, so there may not be a family history. About 10% of these sporadic cases are attributed to new mutations and 20% are attributed to mosaicism [2].

The Double Homeobox Protein 4 (DUX4) is the embryonic transcriptional activator responsible for the disease. DUX4 induces changes in the expression of hundreds of genes that impact many interconnected pathways, making a relationship between gene expression and muscle degeneration difficult to discern [2]. Evidence reveals a complex RNA-mediated process that prompts a robust immune attack on myocytes [4]. It is found in embryonic tissues and allows for apoptosis of cells during formation [5–7].

There are two types of FSHD: Type 1 and Type 2. Type 1 results from a contraction of the D4Z4 repeat. Type 2 is due to mutations in silencing proteins. Both cases lead to chromatin relaxation and aberrant expression of the DUX4 gene in skeletal muscle [8]. The entire D4Z4 region is normally hypermethylated (and therefore silenced), but FSHD is characterized by hypomethylation of D4Z4. There are also two polymorphic genes (4qA and 4qB) that are also required to produce the disease. 4qA has the ability to be pathogenic and 4qB does not, so at least one 4qA allele is required to produce FSHD [2].

The 4qA allele contains a promoter region pLAM, which allows for the DUX4 protein to be transcribed. The 4qB allele lacks pLAM, so the protein cannot be produced. Since there are two copies of chromosome 4 in a cell; AA, BB, or AB are possible, but the presence of at least one A allele is required to produce FSHD, regardless of the presence of Type 1 or Type 2 mutations. This makes FSHD a digenic disease, as two mutations are required to produce disease (A-allele plus Type 1 or Type 2 mutations) [8].

2.1 Type 1 FSHD

Type 1 FSHD affects 95% of FSHD patients. It is caused by shortening of the D4Z4 array, which leads to hypomethylation and chromatin relaxation. The D4Z4 array is a 3300 DNA base pair (3.3 kb) long repeat units on the long arm (q) of chromosome 4. Subtelomeric regions of 4q and 10q at both 4q35 and 10q26 contain D4Z4 arrays, but only the locus at 4q35 results in FSHD [8]. There can be 1–100 units of the D4Z4 repeat. FSHD is associated with an array of 1–10 units at 4q35, although cases with 11 or slightly greater have been described. Patients carrying 1–3 units are usually severely affected and often represent new mutations, while patients carrying 4–10 units are typically familial cases [9]. There is an approximate inverse relationship of residual repeat size to the severity of the disease and the age at onset. A high degree of variability of disease expression even in patients with fragments of the same size makes it impossible to predict disease severity and progression in a given individual based on genetics alone.

2.2 Type 2 FSHD

Type 2 FSHD affects 5% of FSHD patients. It is usually caused by a mutation in the epigenetic modifier gene SMCHD1 on chromosome 18, but 20% of FSHD2 patients do not have an identified mutation in the SMCHD1 gene, so the cause of the hypomethylation is unknown. SMCHD1 provides instructions for making a protein that normally hypermethylates the D4Z4 region. A mutation in this gene leads to haploinsufficiency or dominant negative mutations in SMCDH1 protein, leading to a reduced binding of SMCHD1 protein to the D4Z4 repeat and consequently to a loss of epigenetic marks (methylation) in this region. Some patients with Type 1 mutation can also have a Type 2 mutation, which worsens the disease [10].

3. Clinical manifestations

There is a high degree of variability in phenotype. FSHD1 and FSHD2 are clinically indistinguishable. Patients present most frequently with the inability to lift arms overhead (82%) in the second or third decade of life. About 10% of patients notice facial weakness first, 8% of patients notice ankle dorsiflexion weakness first, and 5% notice pelvic girdle weakness first (these patients are often confused with Limb Girdle Muscular Dystrophy patients). Typically, facial, shoulder, and arm muscles are involved. Facial muscles, including orbicularis oculi and orbicularis oris with asymmetric involvement around the lips can occur. The mechanism of the asymmetry is unknown. Orofacial dysphagia without atrophy of the pharyngeal muscles can also occur. On MRI, tongue atrophy can be seen. The serratus anterior and rhomboids in the shoulder girdle (scapulo-) as well as biceps and triceps in the upper arms (humeral) are commonly involved. There is a lack of contractures around the weak muscles, which is often found in other forms of muscular dystrophy, such as Emery Dreyfus [9].

FSHD typically progresses from the upper to lower extremities. In the lower extremities, it progresses distal (TA, gastrocnemius) to proximal (quadriceps, hamstrings). There is involvement of the core muscles in an asymmetric pattern, including paraspinal muscles and abdominal muscles, leading to lumbar lordosis or camptocormia. The need for wheelchair occurs in 20% of patients in a bimodal distribution. In the severe infantile form with one to three D4Z4 units, the need for a wheelchair occurs in the second decade of life [9]. In other forms, it usually occurs when the patient is over age 50.

A Dutch study of 18% of their FSHD population showed that 74% of patients experienced pain for more than 4 days a month and 58% experienced pain for 4 or more days per week [9]. A French study showed that the cause of pain seemed to be exertion in 91% of patients or faulty posture due to weakness in 74% of patients [9]. Environmental temperature seemed to be a factor in 48% and humidity was a factor in 27% of patients. Pain management techniques, including analgesics, hot baths or showers, and massage provided only temporary relief. About 61% of patients report severe fatigue.

In the infantile form, large deletions resulting in fragments of only one to three D4Z4 repeats occur. Early onset cases are usually sporadic and are occasionally diagnosed as Möbius syndrome. A Japanese study found an association with mental retardation and epilepsy in people with an early onset who are severely affected, although FSHD patients are usually mentally and cognitively normal [11].

3.1 Examination findings

Facial weakness is found in 94% of patients and is demonstrated by decreased brow furrow, inability to close their eyes fully or bury their eyelashes, or the inability to tense their platysma. In the chest wall, examination may reveal pectoral wasting, an exaggerated or inverted axillary crease, and 5% of patients will have pectus excavatum. Shoulder girdle weakness occurs in 93% of cases and may be demonstrated by flattening of clavicular angle, rounding of shoulders, internal rotation of arms or triple hump sign (**Figure 1**), which is alternating muscle and bony landmarks on arm and shoulder. In the arms, one can see Popeye arm with wasting of biceps and triceps muscles and preservation of distal forearm muscles until late in disease. In the back, there is often lateral winging of the scapula with shoulder abduction or flexion (**Figure 2**). About 67% have ankle dorsiflexion weakness and 50% have pelvic girdle weakness. Patients often have a protuberant abdomen with demonstration of Beevor sign (**Figure 3**), which is asymmetric rise in umbilicus with abdominal tensing [2].

3.2 Cardiorespiratory involvement

About 0–13% of patients have restrictive lung disease due to loss of core strength. One percent of patients in a Dutch study were on nocturnal ventilatory support [12]. Risk factors for respiratory compromise include severe disease with wheelchair confinement, moderate to severe kyphoscoliosis, and presence of pectus excavatum.

Cardiomyopathy is not typical, although preclinical reduction of left ventricular function has been described. Asymptomatic supraventricular arrhythmias occur in ~12% [12]. One study showed one-third of their subjects had right bundle branch block that did not progress over 8 years [12].

3.3 Ocular findings

Orbicularis oculi weakness causes incomplete lid closure (lagophthalmos), can lead to exposure keratitis and corneal scarring [2]. Eye drops, ointments, taping, or patches are not always successful in managing these problems. Peripheral telangiectasias of the retina occur in up to one-fourth of patients. Coats disease is an eye disease that can lead to retinal detachment and blindness. Although it usually occurs in males and is unilateral, in FSHD, it occurs in females and is bilateral. Coats disease affects less than 1% of FSHD patients and more commonly affects those with the smallest number of units (one to three D4Z4 units).

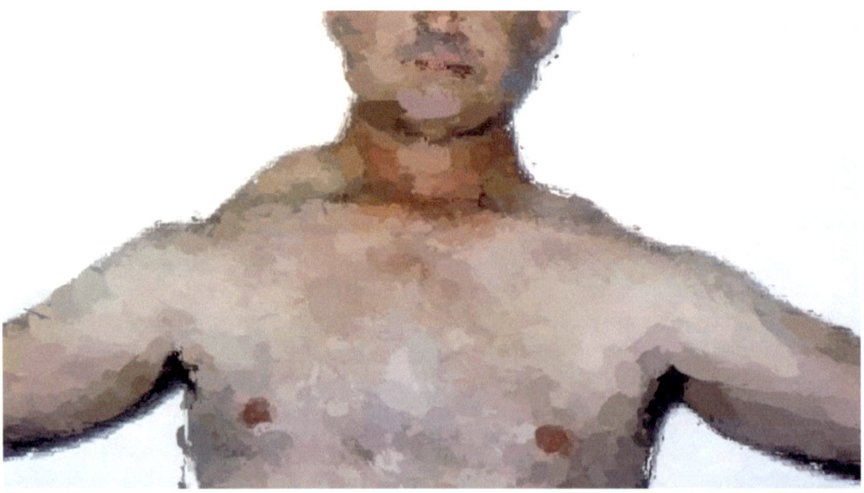

Figure 1.
Triple hump sign: Alternating muscle and bony landmarks of shoulder girdle muscles. Source: Muscular Dystrophy Association.

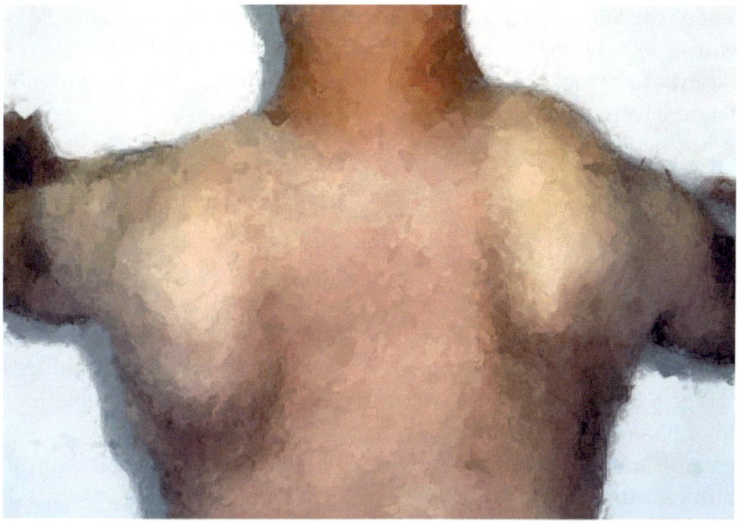

Figure 2.
Winged scapula (right). Source: Muscular Dystrophy Association.

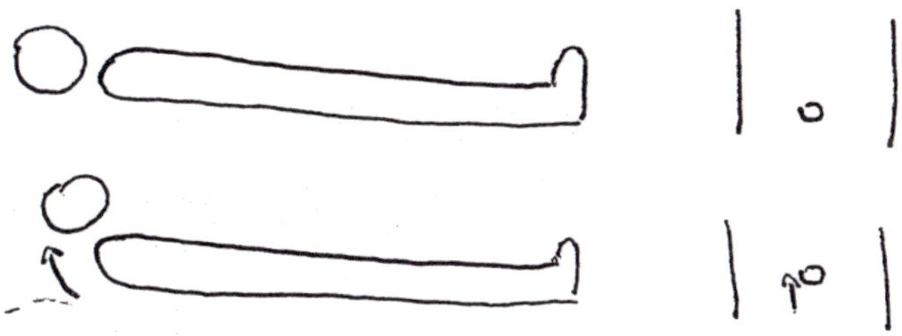

Figure 3.
Beevor sign: When the patients lift their head, their umbilicus displaces up and to the side.

3.4 Ear findings

Asymptomatic loss of high-frequency hearing occurs in up to 65% of patients [2]. Hearing loss, requiring hearing aids affects patients with the smallest number of units (one to four D4Z4 units).

4. Diagnostic testing

Current guidelines call for genetic testing in all patients with clinical FSHD [2]. Labs that perform genetic testing for FSHD first test for D4Z4 contraction using a Southern blot, which has a sensitivity of 93% and specificity of 98%. Normal patients have fragments over 38 kb, but patients with FSHD1 have fragments 10–38 kb, corresponding to 1–10 residual D4Z4 units. If this is negative, then the lab will determine if there is at least one A allele and less than 20% methylation to confirm FSHD2. Genetic testing for SMCHD1 gene is available; however the gene will only be expressed in a low methylation environment [8].

EMG shows small polyphasic motor units (myopathic units) with positive sharp waves or fibrillations. Muscle biopsy shows variation in fiber size, internal myonuclei, degenerating and regenerating myofibers, and increased fibrosis or fatty replacement of muscle. About 5–30% also show perivascular inflammatory infiltrate, consisting of CD4 or CD8 cells. CK is modestly elevated at less than 10 times the upper limit of normal [2]. An MRI of the thigh shows hamstring involvement more than quadriceps involvement [9].

5. Treatment

Currently, there is no cure for FSHD. Scapulopexy (fascial or synthetic slings are used to improve scapular fixation to the thorax) or scapulodesis (scapula is fixed to the thoracic wall to produce a solid fusion) resulted in significant improvement in function, according to one study. Improvements were measured by ability to abduct the shoulder at 1 year and by patient-perceived improvement in the performance of activities of daily living [13].

Conservative management of FSHD includes referral to speech therapy for compensatory strategies for swallowing, ophthalmology consultation for eye issues, periodic hearing screenings, yearly EKGs, physical therapy, and occupational therapy and bracing. Abdominal supports and binders are useful for truncal weakness. The braces most commonly recommended for foot drop include fixed or hinged ankle-foot orthoses or floor reaction orthoses [9].

A Cochrane review of strength training and aerobic exercise training for muscle disease concluded that moderate-intensity strength training does not produce any benefit or harm in patients with FSHD [14].

5.1 New treatment literature review

5.1.1 Losmapimod

Researchers looked into preventing expression of DUX4 mRNA [15]. Past research showed agonists of the β-2 adrenergic receptor suppress DUX4 expression by activating adenylate cyclase to increase cAMP levels. In vitro experiments demonstrate that clinically advanced p38 inhibitors suppress DUX4 expression in FSHD type 1 and 2 myoblasts. Individual small interfering RNA-mediated knockdown of either p38α or p38β suppresses DUX4 expression. p38 inhibitors effectively suppress DUX4 expression in a mouse xenograft model of human FSHD gene regulation. These data support the repurposing of existing clinical p38 inhibitors as potential therapeutics for FSHD.

p38α and p38β isoforms each independently contribute to DUX4 expression, so p38 isoform-selective inhibitors may balance efficacy and safety in skeletal muscle.

Losmapimod inhibits enzymes p38α/β mitogen-activated protein kinases (MAPKs). It has the drawback that p38 kinase inhibition could impair myogenesis by impairing myotube formation. However, GlaxoSmithKline clinical trials showed that losmapimod was generally well tolerated in over 3500 subjects. Two clinical trials of losmapimod for treatment of FSHD are going on at the time this chapter was written. ReDUX4 is evaluating drug efficacy in a randomized controlled phase IIb clinical trial with an estimated study completion date of August 2020. A phase II open-label clinical trial in the Netherlands, with an estimated study completion date of January 2021 is also ongoing at the time this chapter was written.

5.1.2 Resolaris

ATYR1940 (Resolaris) is based on a protein naturally secreted from muscle (resokine) that may act to decrease T-cell activation against muscle [16]. Quality of life and muscle strength of patients treated with Resolaris improved compared to those on placebo, as assessed by individualized neuromuscular quality of life (INQoL) and manual muscle testing (MMT) scores. The phase 1/2 trial was completed in March of 2017. Results showed no significant trend of worsening in MMT or INQoL assessment scores. However, there was a low sample size of nine with three drop outs. The results of a phase 1b/2 trial of 18 patients with LGMD2B and FSHD showed that Resolaris did not suppress circulating immune cells and muscle function by MMT at 14 weeks improved in 50% of FSHD patients. Participants maintained or increased their MMT and INQoL scores at 24 and 36 weeks.

5.1.3 Decoy nucleic acid

A patented decoy nucleic acid can inhibit DUX4-mediated gene activation by binding to the DNA-binding site of the DUX4 transcription factor protein [17]. AAV vectors carrying in their genome two DUX4-binding sites injected in TA muscles of mice also receiving a DUX4-coding plasmid via electron transfer. In a study, AAV carrying the decoy oligonucleotide (AAV D3) significantly decreases DUX4 target gene (mTm7sf4) expression as compared to a control AAV. They concluded that AAV with a DUX4 decoy can inhibit DUX4 expression, making it a future treatment possibility for FSHD patients. DUX4 mRNAs observed in muscle and stem cells are heterogeneous, which can make targeting difficult.

5.1.4 Antisense oligonucleotides

The use of antisense oligonucleotides (AOs) targeting the DUX4 mRNA may interfere either with transcript cleavage/polyadenylation or intron splicing [18]. DUX4-targeted ASOs suppressed the atrophic FSHD myotube phenotype. The ASOs were not shown to improve the disorganized FSHD myotube phenotype, which could be caused by DUX4c over-expression. Therefore, DUX4c might constitute another therapeutic target in FSHD.

5.1.5 Electrical stimulation

In a French study, electrical stimulation was performed to stimulate weak muscles with the goal of strengthening them [19]. They used an HVPG stimulator (Elettronica Pagani, Performer 982, Class Type BF, S/N:181, 2004, Supplier: Libor Medical Products, Ankara/Turkey, Manufacturer: Medical Expo Paderno Dugnano, Italy), using monophasic wave type (twin peak pulse) via surface electrodes. The pulse frequency of the device was 2–100 Hz, voltage output was 0–500 V, and pulse duration was 200 μs. They used a pulse frequency of 50 Hz for optimal contraction. Four electrodes were placed around the muscle and current intensity was increased up to significant contraction. Duty cycle was set at 5 seconds on and 10 seconds off, during 10 minutes of stimulation of each muscle. This was applied 3 times a week, for 8 weeks. Electrostimulation was effective in increasing the strengths of the deltoid and quadriceps femoris muscles. Muscle strength of the deltoid was higher in the electrical stimulation group, and the difference between the groups was maintained in the follow-up period ($p < 0.05$). Additionally, the electrical stimulation group presented more obvious overall improvements than the exercise therapy group according to muscle strength, endurance, and timed performance tests.

5.1.6 Ace-083

ACE-083 binds to and inhibits select proteins in the TGF-beta protein superfamily, namely activins and myostatin, which reduce muscle growth [20]. If a person stops exercising, the muscles gradually reduce in size, due to the function of activins and myostatin, among other factors. Inhibiting the TGF-beta family reduces or slows this muscle breakdown. The researchers looked into whether this can be helpful for patients with Charcot–Marie-Tooth (CMT) or FSHD. However, phase 2 clinical trials showed a lack of efficacy, so Acceleron halted the development of ACE-083 for FSHD. Trials for CMT were not halted.

6. Conclusion

Facioscapulohumeral muscular dystrophy is a disease with no cure; however, current research is promising for a cure in the near future. Technologies in genetic editing show particular promise in the field of muscular dystrophy. Molecular mechanisms of genetic diseases, even those with known mechanisms, are oftentimes much more complex than initially thought. Discoveries regarding transcription modulators have proven particularly useful in research to find treatments for muscular dystrophies. Given recent advances in these areas, the future appears bright for patients with muscular dystrophy.

Acknowledgements

The author would like to thank the Muscular Dystrophy Association for their support and acknowledge Dr. Dale Lange for inspiring the author's interest in neuromuscular medicine.

My program director, Dr. Dora Leung, was instrumental in defining the path of the author's career. For this, the author is extremely grateful.

Conflict of interest

The author declares no conflict of interest.

Author details

Robin Warner
Department of Neurology, Hospital for Special Surgery, New York, USA

*Address all correspondence to: warnerr@hss.edu

References

[1] Teveroni E et al. Estrogens enhance myoblast differentiation in facioscapulohumeral muscular dystrophy by antagonizing DUX4 activity. The Journal of Clinical Investigation. 2017;**127**(4):1531-1545. DOI: 10.1172/JCI89401

[2] Stratland JM, Tawil R. Facioscapulohumeral Muscular Dystrophy. Continuum. 2016;**22**(6):1917-1931. DOI: 10.1212/CON.0000000000000399

[3] Tawil R, McDermott MP, Mendell JR, et al. FSHD: Design of natural history study and results of baseline testing. Neurology. 1994;**44**:442-446

[4] Shadle SC et al. DUX4-induced dsRNA and MYC mRNA stabilization activate apoptotic pathways in human cell models of facioscapulohumeral dystrophy. PLoS Genetics. 2017;**13**(3):e1006658. DOI: 10.1371/journal.pgen.1006658

[5] Whiddon JL et al. Conservation and innovation in the DUX4-family gene network. Nature Genetics. 2017;**49**(6):935-940. DOI: 10.1038/ng.3846. [Epub: 01 May 2017]

[6] Hendrickson PG et al. Conserved roles of mouse DUX and human DUX4 in activating cleavage-stage genes and MERVL/HERVL retrotransposons. Nature Genetics. 2017;**49**(6):925-934

[7] De Iaco A et al. DUX-family transcription factors regulate zygotic genome activation in placental mammals. Nature Genetics. 2017;**49**(6):941-945

[8] Tawil R, Van Der Maarel SM. Facioscapulohumeral muscular dystrophy. Muscle and Nerve. 2006;**34**:1-15

[9] Pandya S, King WM, Tawil R. Facioscapulohumeral dystrophy. Physical Therapy. 2008;**88**(1):105-113. DOI: 10.2522/ptj.20070104

[10] Mason AG et al. SMCHD1 regulates a limited set of gene clusters on autosomal chromosomes. Skeletal Muscle. 2017;**7**(1):12. DOI: 10.1186/s13395-017-0129-7

[11] Funakoshi M, Goto K, Arahata K. Epilepsy and mental retardation in a subset of early onset 4q35-facioscapulohumeral muscular dystrophy. Neurology. 1998;**50**(6):1791-1794. DOI: 10.1212/wnl.50.6.1791

[12] van Dijk GP, van der Kooi E, Begin A, et al. High prevalence of incomplete right bundle branch block in facioscapulohumeral muscular dystrophy without cardiac symptoms. Functional Neurology. 2014;**29**(3):159-165

[13] Orrell RW, Copeland S, Rose MR. Scapular fixation in muscular dystrophy. Cochrane Database of Systematic Reviews. 2010;(1). Artical number: CD003278. DOI: 10.1002/14651858.CD003278.pub2

[14] van der Kooi EL, Lindeman E, Riphagen I. Strength training and aerobic exercise training for muscle disease. Cochrane Database of Systematic Reviews. 2005;**1**:CD003907

[15] Oliva J, Galasinski S, Richey A, Campbell AE, Meyers MJ, Modi N, et al. Clinically advanced p38 inhibitors suppress DUX4 expression in cellular and animal models of facioscapulohumeral muscular dystrophy. The Journal of Pharmacology and Experimental Therapeutics. 2019. DOI: 10.1124/jpet.119.259663

[16] Gershman A, Chiang K, Do M, Abbink E, Harbers V, Audebert C,

et al. A randomized, double-blinded, placebo-controlled, multiple ascending dose study to evaluate the safety, tolerability, pharmacokinetics, immunogenicity, and biological activity of ATYR1940 in adult patients with facioscapulohumeral muscular dystrophy (FSHD). Neuromuscular Disorders. 2016;**26**(Supplement 2):S167. DOI: 10.1016/j.nmd.2016.06.293

[17] Dumonceaux J, Voit T, Mariot V. Treatment of Facioscapulohumeral Dystrophy. 2019. Available from: http://www.freepatentsonline.com/y2018/0016577.html

[18] Ansseau E, Vanderplanck C, Belayew A. Antisense oligonucleotides used to target the DUX4 mRNA as therapeutic approaches in facioscapulohumeral muscular dystrophy (FSHD). Genes (Basel). 2017;**8**(3):93. DOI: 10.3390/genes8030093

[19] Kilinç M, Yildirim SA, Tan E. The effects of electrical stimulation and exercise therapy in patients with limb girdle muscular dystrophy: A controlled clinical trial. Neurosciences. 2015;**20**(3):259-266. DOI: 10.17712/nsj.2015.3.201501097

[20] Statland J, Bravver E, Karam C, Elman L, Johnson N, Joyce N, et al. Results for a dose-escalation phase 2 study to evaluate ACE-083, a local muscle therapeutic, in patients with facioscapulohumeral muscular dystrophy. Neuromuscular Disorders. 2018;**28**(Supplement 2):S140. DOI: 10.1016/j.nmd.2018.06.413

Chapter 3

miRNAs and Muscle Stem Cells

Francisco Hernandez-Torres, Lara Rodriguez-Outeiriño, Lidia Matias-Valiente, Estefania Lozano-Velasco, Diego Franco and Amelia Aranega

Abstract

Skeletal muscle represents between 30 and 38% of the human body mass. Both the maintenance and repair of adult muscle tissue are directed by satellite cells (SCs). SCs are located beneath the basal lamina of the skeletal muscle myofiber. They are quiescent for most of their life but, in response to physiological stimuli or muscle trauma, they activate, proliferate, and enter the myogenic program via generating myogenic progenitors (myoblasts) that fuse to existing myofibers or *de novo* myofibers. MicroRNAs (miRNAs or miRs) play a critical role in regulating muscle regeneration and stem cell behavior. In this chapter, we review the pivotal role in the regulation of SC quiescence, activation, and differentiation in the context of muscular dystrophies.

Keywords: microRNA, satellite cell, quiescence, myogenesis, muscle regeneration, muscular dystrophies

1. Introduction

With more than 600 individual muscles in humans, skeletal muscle tissue represents between 30 and 38% of the human body mass [1]. This tissue is essential not only to provide ambulatory capacity to our organism but also to control such important functions as breathing and thermogenesis. Although its composition is heterogenous, each single skeletal muscle is mainly composed by individual muscle fibers consisting of elongated multinucleated syncytia. These myofibers are diversified in size, shape, and contractile protein content to fulfill the different functional needs of our body. This tissue retains a highly adaptive and robust capacity to regenerate throughout most of life, thanks to the presence of a stem cell-like population termed as satellite cells (SCs) [2].

miRNAs have emerged as critical regulators of numerous biological processes by modulating gene expression at the posttranscriptional level. The discovery of *miRNAs* as new and important regulators of gene expression is expected to broaden our biological understanding of the regulatory mechanism in muscle by adding another dimension of regulation to the diversity and complexity of gene regulatory networks. In that context, the role of *miRNAs* in SC biology is beginning to be explored. In this chapter, we will focus in our understanding of how miRNAs act in controlling the ability of SCs to appropriately balance SC function during muscle regeneration as well as in the context of neuromuscular diseases.

2. Basic biology of SCs

SCs, originally identified via electron microscopy in 1961 by Alexander Mauro, are located underneath the basal lamina and adjacent to the plasma membrane of the skeletal muscle myofiber [3]. It has been established that SCs in adult muscle represent a lineage continuum of embryonic myogenic progenitor cells. SCs of the body and limbs arise from somites, in common with the muscle that they are associated with [4–6], while SCs located in head muscles also originate from the cranial mesoderm [7]. In undamaged muscle, the majority of *satellite cells* are *quiescent*, characterized by the expression of the transcription factor PAX7 [8]. Within a context of physiological stimuli (physical exercise or pathological conditions), SCs become activated and enter into the cell cycle to expand their progeny and form myogenic precursor cells or myoblasts [8]. SCs' activation is mediated by the induced expression of myogenic factor 5 (MYF5) and myogenic determination protein (MYOD) [2]. The differentiation of myogenic committed cells involves downregulation of PAX7 and *de novo* expression of myogenin (MYOG), which is followed by fusion of the newly formed differentiated myoblasts among them and with the remaining myofibers to repair damaged muscle [2]. In addition to providing myogenic precursors, activated SCs also undergo self-renewing proliferation that replenishes the pool of muscle SCs, thereby ensuring that the capacity to respond to future injuries is maintained in the muscle [2].

3. Biogenesis of miRNAs

Canonical miRNAs are transcribed by RNA polymerase II into primary transcripts called pri-miRNA, bearing 5′m7G cap and 3′ poly(A) tail structures [9]. Sometimes, miRNA loci can comprise no single but multiple and overlapping miRNA genes, called clusters, which are processed from the same polycistronic primary transcript [10]. Once transcribed, the pri-miRNA forms a stem-loop structure. Then, the RNA-binding protein Di George syndrome critical region gene 8 (DGCR8) recognizes it and directs the nuclear RNase III enzyme endonuclease, DROSHA, toward the pri-miRNA. DROSHA cleaves at the base of the hairpin embedded within the pri-miRNA [11], yielding a ~70-nt hairpin molecule termed precursor miRNA or pre-miRNA. Soon after, the pre-miRNA is transported from the nucleus by exportin 5 to the cytoplasm via a Ran-GTP-dependent mechanism [12]. Once in the cytoplasm, a second RNase III endonuclease, DICER, cleaves the pre-miRNA, thus removing the terminal loop of the pre-miRNA and releasing a mature double-stranded ~22-nt miRNA molecule [13]. One strand of this duplex RNA molecule (the guide strand) is transferred to the RNA-induced silencing complex (RISC) containing argonaute 2 (AGO2) and the RNA-binding protein TARBP2 [TAR (HIV) RNA-binding protein 2], while the other is degraded [14]. The miRNA's function at this time is to guide the silencing complex to the target mRNA through complementary binding of the miRNA seed sequence, which results in inhibition of translation and/or degradation of the target transcript [15] (**Figure 1**).

Approximately, half of vertebrate miRNAs are processed from introns of protein-coding genes or genes encoding for other ncRNA classes, for instance, small nucleolar RNA (snoRNAs) or long intervening noncoding RNAs (lincRNAs) [10]. The biosynthesis of these miRNAs bypass one or more steps in the canonical biogenesis pathway, being therefore termed noncanonical miRNAs. In this sense, it is important to stress that while DROSHA and DGCR8 are only needed to process canonical miRNAs, DICER is almost always indispensable in the production of both canonical and noncanonical miRNAs [16]. Among noncanonical miRNAs, the most

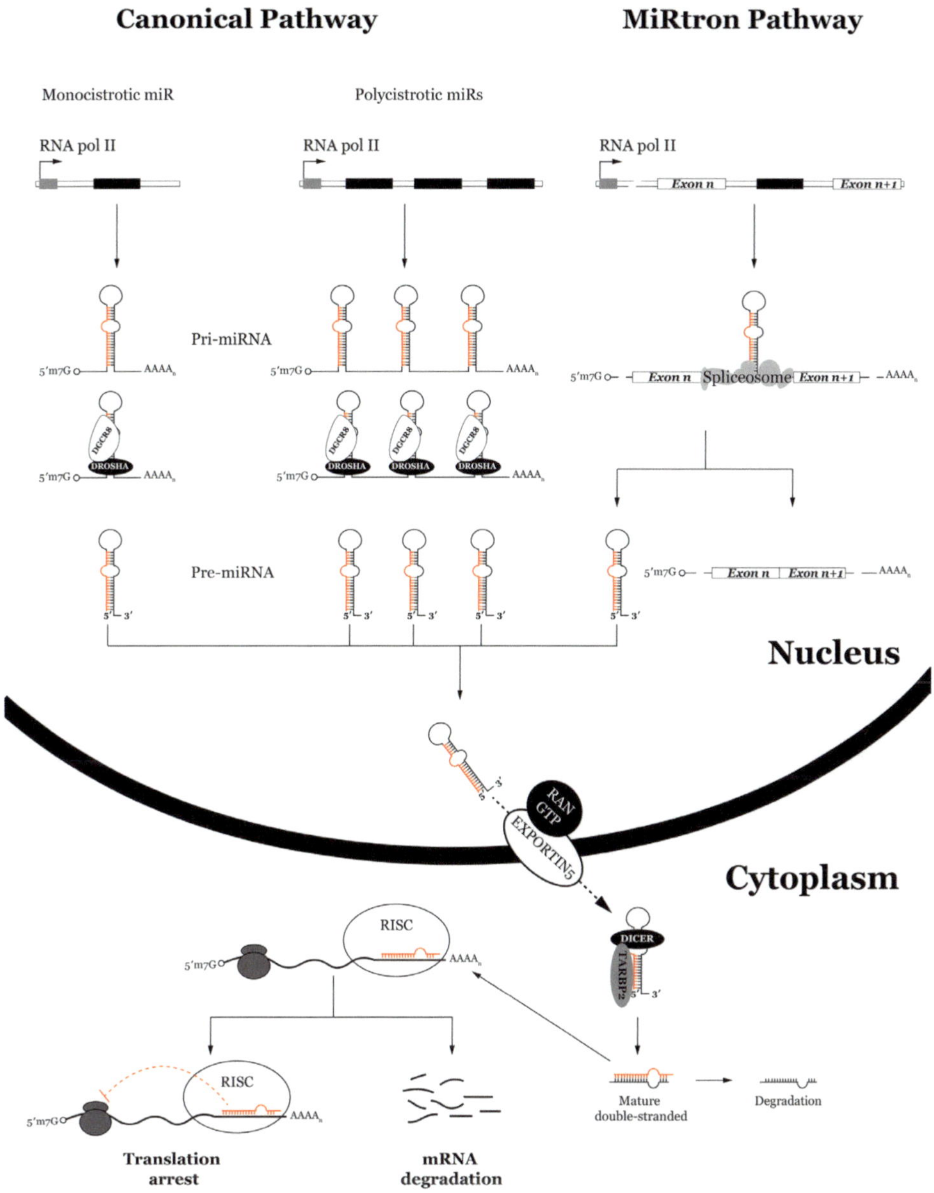

Figure 1.
Schematic representation of biogenesis of miRNAs.

studied have been those so-called miRtrons, located within intron sequences. The expression profiles of these miRNAs coincide with the transcription of their host genes [10], being released from the excised host introns by the spliceosome [17, 18] in a typical mirtron-maturing fashion (**Figure 1**).

4. miRNAs and SC function

Deep sequencing analyses have shown that many miRs are expressed in muscle tissue [19–21]. Among these miRs, there is a group, so-called myomiRs, whose expression is restricted to muscle tissue. This family is composed by miR-1, miR-133a, and miR-206, miR208a, miR-208b, miR-486, and miR-499 [22–28]. While most myomiR family members are expressed in both the heart and skeletal muscle, miR-208a is cardiac-specific and miR-206 is skeletal muscle-specific. A deeper analysis of these family members is well reviewed in [29]. Nevertheless, not only myomiRs but also other miRs with a more ubiquitous expression play important roles in the muscle. It has also been shown that miRNAs are essential for muscle homeostasis and regeneration upon injury, since either systemic or conditional deletion of DICER in muscle $PAX7^+$ population results in a depletion of SCs and a quasi-absence of repair upon injury cell [30]. In addition, to date, *in vitro* and *in vivo* experiments have shown that many miRs expressed in the skeletal muscle rule quiescence, activation, proliferation, fate specification, and differentiation of muscle progenitor cells by regulating the expression of myogenic differentiation regulators, transcription factors, structural proteins, and cytoskeletal components that are required to give rise to the differentiated muscle phenotype. In this section, we will review some of them, analyzing their roles in quiescence, activation-proliferation, and differentiation estates.

4.1 Control of the quiescence state

In vivo, SCs are normally in a quiescent state after the postnatal development. Cheung et al. showed that the quiescent state is strongly controlled by miRs, since SCs lacking a functional *Dicer* gene, spontaneously exit from the quiescent state [30]. In this work, the authors demonstrate that miR-489 regulates SCs quiescence in a cell-autonomous manner through the control of the oncogene *Dek* (DEK proto-oncogene), whose protein is not expressed in quiescent SCs (QSCs) but is strongly upregulated after SC activation. Soon after, Crist et al. showed that miR-31 targets *Myf5* mRNA in QSCs, thus preventing MYF5 protein accumulation and premature activation of these muscle stem cells [31]. miR-31 is sequestered with *Myf5* transcripts in cytoplasmic mRNP granules in QSCs and, upon SCs' activation, these mRNPs rapidly dissociate and relieve the spatial constraint on miR-31 and Myf5 mRNA, allowing the rapid translation of the MYF5 protein. Recently, Baghdadi et al. have added a new miR to the list of miRs that control the quiescent state of SCs [32]. In this work, the authors shown that miR-708 regulates quiescence and self-renewal by active repression of SC migration. Notch signaling is directly implicated in this control by inducing transcription of miR-708 that represses Tensin3 (*Tns3*), a component of the focal adhesion complex. This repression inhibits focal adhesion kinase (FAK) activation, which in turn stabilizes SCs within their niche (**Table 1** and **Figure 2**).

4.2 Activated proliferative state

Early evidences of miRs controlling proliferation in myoblast were reported by Chen et al. in 2006 [33]. In this work, the authors showed that miR-133 enhances myoblast proliferation by repressing the serum response factor (Srf) *in vitro* and *in vivo* in *Xenopus laevis* embryos. Similarly, Cai et al. have recently shown that miR-664 also promotes myoblast proliferation by targeting *Srf* mRNA [34]. Other miR that proposed to promote myoblast proliferation is miR-27. Huang et al. showed that miR-27, for this purpose, targets myostatin (Mstn), a well-known negative regulator of myogenesis [35]. Sometimes, miR members of a same cluster can work together in order to achieve the same biological effect. In this sense, Qiu et al. have shown that miR-17, miR-20a, and miR-92a, three members of the miR-17-92 cluster, repress PDZ and LIM domain 5 (Pdlim5), also known as Enh1 expression at heart and skeletal muscle. This protein exerts antiproliferative effects in myoblast. Thus, its inhibition contributes to promote myoblast proliferation and prevents differentiation [36] (**Table 1** and **Figure 2**).

microRNAs	Targets	Function	References
miR-489	*Dek*	Regulates SCs' quiescence	[30]
miR-31	*Myf5*	Prevents MYF5 protein accumulation and premature activation of SCs	[31]
miR-708	*Tns3*	Regulates quiescence and self-renewal by active repression of SCs' migration	[32]
miR-133	*Srf*	Enhances and/or promotes myoblast proliferation	[33]
miR-664	*Srf*	Enhances and/or promotes myoblast proliferation	[34]
miR-27	*Mstn*	Enhances and/or promotes myoblast proliferation	[35]
miR-17, miR-20a, and miR-92a	*Pdlim5*	Enhance and/or promotes myoblast proliferation	[36]
miR-195 and miR-497	*Igf1r, Insr, Ccne1, and Ccnd2*	Inhibit myoblast proliferation	[37]
miR-487b	*Irs1*	Inhibits myoblast proliferation	[38]
miR-16	*Foxo1*	Suppresses myogenesis	[39]
miR-1 and miR-133	*Ccnd1 and Sp1*	Inhibit myoblast proliferation	[40]
miR-15b, miR-23b, miR-106b, and miR-503	*Ccnd1 and Ccnd2*	Keep SCs in a quiescent state	[41]
miR-106b	*Myf5*	Keeps SCs in a quiescent state	[41]
miR-1	*Hdac4*	Promotes myoblast differentiation	[33]
miR-1 and miR-206	*Pax7*	Restrict myogenic progenitor cell proliferation and promote differentiation	[42]
miR-206	*Pax7*	Activates myoblast differentiation	[43]
miR-206	*Pax7, Notch3, and Igfbp5*	Stimulates SC differentiation and skeletal muscle regeneration	[44]
miR-206	*Hdac4 and Pola1*	Promotes myoblast differentiation and induces a cell cycle arrest	[45]
miR-1 and miR-206	*Gja1*	Promote myoblast fusion	[46]
miR-206 and miR-486	*Pax7*	Promote initial muscle differentiation	[47]
miR-486	*Pten, Pdgfrβ, Foxo1, Sfrs1, and Sfrs3*	Promotes myoblast differentiation	[48–50]
miR-133	*Fgfr1 and Pp2ac*	Promotes muscle precursor cells differentiation	[51]
miR-29	*Rybp and Yy1*	Ensures proper myoblast differentiation into myotubes	[52]
miR-29	*Hdac4*	Promotes myoblast differentiation	[53]
miR-29	*Akt3*	Reduces proliferation and facilitates differentiation of precursor muscle cells	[54]
miR-26a	*Ezh2*	Induces muscle cell differentiation	[55]
miR-26a	*Smad1 and Smad4*	Promotes myoblast differentiation	[56]
miR-214	*Ezh2*	Promotes myoblast differentiation	[57]
miR-214	*N-ras*	Promotes myogenic differentiation by facilitating exit from mitosis	[58]

microRNAs	Targets	Function	References
miR-181	*HoxA11*	Promotes myogenic differentiation	[59]
miR-378	*MyoR*	Promotes myogenic differentiation	[60]
miR-205a	*Cdh11*	Inhibits myoblast proliferation and promotes myoblast differentiation	[61]
MiR-675-3p	*Smad1 and Smad5*	Promotes myogenic differentiation by repression of BMP pathway	[62]
miR-675-5p	*Cdc6*	Promotes myogenic differentiation by repression of DNA replication	[62]
miR-17	*Ccnd2, Jak1, and Rhoc*	Promotes differentiation of precursor muscle cells	[63]
miR-34b	*Igfbp2*	Represses proliferation and promotes differentiation of myoblasts	[64]
miR-664	*Wnt1*	Downregulates WNT signaling to allow for normal myogenic differentiation to occur	[34]
miR-199a	*Wnt2, Fzd4, and Jag1*	Downregulates WNT signaling to allow for normal myogenic differentiation to occur	[65]
miR-155	*Mef2a*	Represses myoblast differentiation	[66]
miR-351	*Lactb*	Represses myoblast differentiation	[67]
miR-23a	*Myh1, Myh2, and Myh4*	Prevents myogenic differentiation	[68]

Table 1.
General overview of miRNAs involved in adult myogenesis.

miRNAs can modulate negative proliferation in myoblast as well. In this sense, Wei et al. showed that the protein complex NF-κB can induce miR-195 and miR-497 expression, thus inhibiting myoblast proliferation by targeting insulin-like growth factor I receptor (Igf1r), insulin receptor (Insr), cyclin E1 (Ccne1), and cyclin D2 (Ccnd2) mRNAs [37]. Thus, NF-κB inhibition must be accomplished to induce proliferation in these cells. Another miR that targets insulin signaling proteins is miR-487b. This miR represses insulin receptor substrate 1 (Irs1) mRNA, thus exerting a negative control of myoblast proliferation [38]. Similarly, it has been reported that miR-16 acts as a coordinated mediator that can suppress myogenesis in avian hypertrophic skeletal muscles through the control of myoblast proliferation by targeting forkhead box O1 (Foxo1) mRNA [39], a transcription factor that governs muscle growth, metabolism, and cell differentiation [69]. Growth factors such as fibroblast growth factors (FGFs) regulate cell proliferation and differentiation in numerous tissues, including skeletal muscle [70]. In this sense, Zhang et al. [40] have shown that FGF2 released from the myotrauma represses p38 signaling and expression of miR-1 and miR-133. Thus, the repressed p38 signaling and subsequent downregulation of miR-1 and 133 induce an upregulation of their respective targets, cyclin D1 (Ccnd1) and Sp1 transcription factor (Sp1), that jointly facilitate the SC proliferation at the early stages of muscle regeneration. Nevertheless, this work contradicts the pro-proliferating role for miR-133 proposed by Chen et al. in 2006 [33]. Our group has also shed light over this issue. Thus, Lozano-Velasco et al. unravel the existence of a Pitx2-miRNA pathway that modulates cell proliferation in myoblasts and skeletal muscle SCs [41]. In this work, we demonstrated that miR-15b, miR-23b, miR-106b, and miR-503 keep SCs in a quiescent state by targeting Ccnd1 and Ccnd2. Once QSCs are activated, Pitx2c is upregulated and exerts a

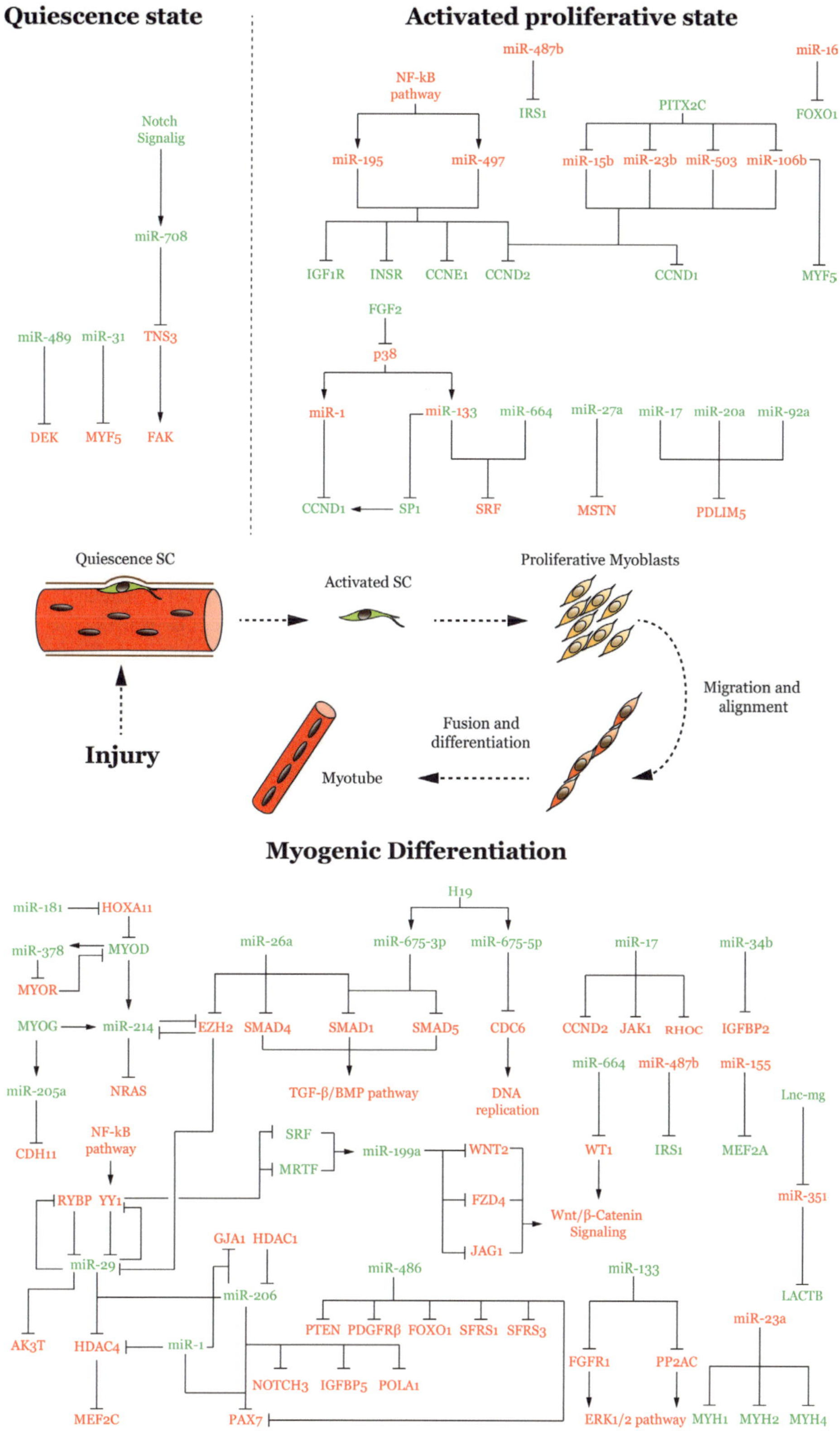

Figure 2.
miR controlling differentiation of muscular precursor cells. Green and red labels correspond with the induced or repressed molecules on each state, respectively (quiescent state, activated proliferative state, or myogenic differentiation).

repressive effect over miR-15b, miR-23b, miR-106b, and miR-503 promoters, thus allowing Ccnd1 and Ccnd2 mRNA to be translated. On the other hand, this Pitx2 upregulation also avoids the repressive effect of miR106b over Myf5 mRNA, thus promoting myoblast commitment to a myogenic cell fate (**Table 1** and **Figure 2**).

4.3 Myogenic differentiation

SC differentiation is a complex process. In this stage, the cells need to switch off proliferative signals and upregulate structural genes turning simple individual cells into a complex syncytium with the ability to coordinately contracts. In this scenario, miRs have also been described as essential molecules. Focusing on myo-miRs, Chen et al. showed that miR-1 promotes myoblast differentiation by targeting histone deacetylase 4 (Hdac4) mRNA, a transcriptional repressor of muscle gene expression [33]. HDAC4 has been shown to inhibit muscle differentiation and skeletal muscle gene expression, mainly by repressing myocyte enhancer factor 2C (MEF2C), an essential muscle-related transcription [71]. The same group also showed that miR-1 and miR-206 restrict myogenic progenitor cell proliferation and promote differentiation by directly downregulating Pax7 expression [42]. At the same time, Cacchiarelli et al. also showed that miR-206 activates myoblast differentiation through Pax7 repression at early stages of differentiation [43]. These authors have shown that, in SCs, miR-206 is specifically repressed by histone deacetylase 1 (HDAC1), but under differentiation conditions, repressive effect over miR-206 promoter mediated by HDAC1 disappear thus allowing Pax7 repression and promoting myoblast differentiation [43]. Soon after, Liu et al. showed that loss of miR-206 results in upregulation of Pax7, notch receptor 3 (Notch3), and insulin-like growth factor-binding protein 5 (Igfbp5) in differentiating miR-206 KO SCs compared with WT cells, implying that repression of these inhibitors of myogenesis accounts, at least in part, for the stimulatory influence of miR-206 on SC differentiation and skeletal muscle regeneration [44]. As miR-1, miR-206 also promotes myoblast differentiation by targeting Hdac4 [53] and induces a cell cycle arrest through the repression of DNA polymerase alpha 1 (Pola1, catalytic subunit), a specific subunit of DNA polymerase α [45]. miR-1 and miR-206 also work coordinately, downregulating gap junction protein (Gja1, alpha also known as Connexin 43) expression during myoblast fusion as Anderson et al. had shown previously [46]. Dey et al. also corroborated that miR-206 targets Pax7 mRNA [47] and, in the same work, they also demonstrated that miR-486 exerts the same effect in order to promote initial muscle differentiation. Regarding this miR, Alexander et al. showed that miR-486 targets phosphatase and tensin homolog (Pten), platelet-derived growth factor receptor beta (Pdgfrβ), Foxo1, serine and arginine-rich splicing factor 1 (Sfrs1), and serine and arginine-rich splicing factor 3 (Sfrs3) mRNAs. Proteins derived from these mRNAs comprise the PTEN/AKT pathway, which is essential for normal cellular proliferation [48–50]. Thus, miR-486 overexpression and consequent PTEN/AKT pathway inhibition are required for proper myoblast differentiation as well. A role for miR-133 in myogenic differentiation has also been proposed. Thus, Feng et al. showed that miR-133 promotes muscle precursor cells differentiation by downregulating two members of the pro-proliferation ERK1/2 signaling pathway, fibroblast growth factor receptor 1 (Fgfr1), and protein phosphatase 2 (Pp2ac, catalytic subunit, alpha isozyme) [51]. All together, these data bring out the important role carried out by myomiRs during early steps of muscle differentiation (**Table 1** and **Figure 2**).

Focusing on non-muscle-specific miRs involved in myogenic differentiation, another miR with a relevant importance during muscle differentiation is miR-29. miR-29 seems to promote myogenesis by downregulating multiple targets related to the NF-kB signaling pathway. In this sense, Wang et al. unraveled a myogenic circuit that involves constitutive activity of NF-kB in myoblasts regulating the YY1 transcription factor, which subsequently suppresses the miR-29 promoter activity by recruiting the enhancer of zeste homolog 2 (histone methyltransferase, EZH2) as well as the histone deacetylase protein HDAC1, thus maintaining cells in an undifferentiated state [72]. In this regard, Zhou et al. later showed that miR-29 is able to directly target the RING1- and YY1-binding protein (Rybp) [52]. RYBP is a negative regulator of skeletal myogenesis, which, together with EZH2 and HDAC1, functions as a corepressor of YY1 to silence miR-29 promoter [52]. Thus, as differentiation ensues, downregulation of the NF-kB-YY1 pathway, RYBP, and EZH2 lead to upregulation of miR-29 that in turns further decreases YY1 and Rybp levels to ensure proper differentiation into myotubes. As miR-1 and miR-206, miR-29 also promotes myoblast differentiation by targeting Hdac4 [53]. In addition, miR-29 targets AKT serine/threonine kinase 3 (Akt3), a member of the serine/threonine protein kinase family responsive to growth factor cell signaling, to reduce proliferation and facilitate differentiation of precursor muscle cells in skeletal muscle development [54] (**Table 1** and **Figure 2**).

Another non-muscle-specific miR whose expression is upregulated during myogenic differentiation is miR-26a. The important role of miR-26 in inducing muscle cell differentiation had also been previously demonstrated by Wong et al., who showed that miR-26 acts to posttranscriptionally repress Ezh2, a known suppressor of skeletal muscle cell differentiation that belongs to the polycomb group (PcG) of proteins that suppress gene transcription through histone methylation, thus promoting miR-29 promoter activity as we have previously indicated [55]. In addition, Dey et al. showed that miR-26a directly targets SMAD family member 1 (Smad1) and SMAD family member 4 (Smad4), two critical transcription factors that belong to TGF-β/BMP pathway, whose activity inhibits myogenesis [56] (**Table 1** and **Figure 2**).

miR-214 upregulation is also required for myogenesis. During SCs' activation and proliferation, EZH2 is highly expressed in the generated myoblasts, thus allowing PcG proteins to repress transcription from the intronic region containing miR-214 [57]. The initial phase of cell differentiation is characterized by reduced Ezh2 expression and consequent derepression of the miR-214 locus. Then, in a negative feedback, miR-214 targets Ezh2 mRNA, thus reducing its translation [57]. At this point, the continuous PcG disengagement leads to recruit MyoD/MyoG to the miR-214 promoter, thus enhancing its transcription [57]. This negative feedback, together with miR-26a via Ezh2, contributes to enhance miR-29 promoter activity. On the other hand, miR-214 is also able to promote myogenic differentiation by facilitating exit from mitosis via downregulation of neuroblastoma ras oncogene (N-ras) [58]. Regarding to the effect that MyoD exerts over miR-214 promoter, Naguibneva et al. demonstrated that homeobox A11 (HoxA11), a negative regulator of MyoD expression, is a direct target of miR-181 during mammalian muscle differentiation. Thus, under differentiation conditions, miR-181 is upregulated, resulting in downregulation of HoxA11 and the consequent release of MyoD expression [59]. MyoD also binds in close proximity to the miR-378 gene and causes its transactivation [60]. Parallelly, this miR targets MyoR mRNA, thus avoiding the antagonist effect of MYOR over MYOD, constituting a feed-forward loop where MyoD indirectly downregulates MyoR via miR-378 [60]. Besides, by using chicken myoblasts, Wang et al. have described how miR-205a is regulated by myogenin (MyoG) transcription factor, which can bind to the promoter region of miR-205a gene in chicken, thus inducing its expression. The upregulation of miR-205a can inhibit myoblast proliferation and promote myoblast differentiation by its repression on cadherin-11 (CDH11), a crucial regulator of postnatal skeletal growth [61] (**Table 1** and **Figure 2**).

H19 long noncoding RNA and its encoded miRNAs, miR-675-3p, and miR-675-5p are expressed in the skeletal muscles and also are upregulated during myoblast differentiation and muscle regeneration [62]. Dey et al. have shown that MiR-675-3p targets Smad1 and SMAD family member 5 (Smad5) mRNAs, while miR-675-5p represses cell division cycle 6 (Cdc6) mRNA. Consequently, through SMAD1 and SMAD5 proteins' downregulation, miR-675-5p induces a repression of BMP pathway as well as a repression of DNA replication through CDC6 protein downregulation, thus promoting myoblast differentiation [62]. Similarly, Kong et al. have also shown that miR-17 targets Ccnd2, Janus kinase 1 (Jak1) and ras homolog family member C (Rhoc) mRNAs. These genes are critical for cell proliferation and/or fusion, hence their inhibition promotes differentiation of precursor muscle cells [63]. In this sense, Wang et al. have also shown that miR-34b represses the proliferation and promotes the differentiation of myoblasts by targeting insulin-like growth factor-binding protein 2 (IGFBP2) [64] (**Table 1** and **Figure 2**).

miR-664 induces myogenic differentiation through targeting Wnt family member 1 (Wnt1), hence blocking the canonical Wnt/β-catenin signaling pathway [34]. In this regard, Alexander et al. unraveled a SRF/MRTF-dependent mechanism for the induction of miR-199a transcription during myoblast differentiation [65]. In this stage, miR-199a represses WNT2, FZD4, and JAG1 and subsequently downregulates WNT signaling to allow for normal myogenic differentiation to occur [65]. In this work, the authors also indicate that, in previous stages, miR-199a-5p transcription is likewise repressed by YY1, as happened with miR29 promoter (**Table 1** and **Figure 2**).

miRNAs can also negatively modulate myoblast differentiation. Thus, it has been shown that miR-487b must be downregulated in order to avoid its suppressive effect over Irs1 mRNA, as happens during proliferation stage [38]. The MEF2 proteins are transcription factors that act in conjunction with myogenic regulatory factors (MRFs) to regulate muscle differentiation [73]. In this sense, Seok et al. showed that miR-155 represses myoblast differentiation by repressing Mef2a mRNA, hence miR-155 downregulation is necessary to prevent Mef2a downregulation and to induce a proper myoblast differentiation [66]. In a newfangled fashion lnc-mg, a long noncoding RNA that promotes myoblast differentiation [74] has been described to act as a competing endogenous RNA (ceRNA) sponging miR-351, thus reducing the effect of miR-351 on its direct target lactamase-β (LACTB) to promote myoblast differentiation [67] (**Table 1** and **Figure 2**).

MiRs are also capable to regulate structural proteins needed at last stages of myoblast differentiation. Regarding this, Wang et al. showed that miR-23a prevents myogenic differentiation through downregulation of fast myosin heavy chain isoforms. Thus, downregulation of miR-23a during final steps of muscle differentiation allows myotubes to express the myosin heavy chain genes Myh1, Myh2, and Myh4 [68] (**Table 1** and **Figure 2**).

5. miRNAs and muscle cells in muscular dystrophies

Primary muscular disorders are the consequence of a disease that directly affects skeletal muscle [75]. Among them, the most important group, in terms of number of people affected as well as economic impact generated in the developed world, are muscular dystrophies. These pathologies are inherited myogenic disorders characterized by progressive muscle wasting and weakness of variable distribution and severity [76]. The genes and their protein products that cause most of these disorders have now been identified [76]. However, miRNAs misregulation related to them still remains poorly understood. In this section, we focus in the understanding of how miRNAs act in regulating muscle cells in the context of Duchenne muscular dystrophy (DMD) and myotonic dystrophy (DM), the most common inherited muscle diseases of childhood and adulthood, respectively. In addition, we discuss current miR-related molecular diagnosis and therapy approaches implemented in the field in order to ameliorate the progression of these pathologies by modulating muscle precursor biology.

5.1 miRNA in muscle precursor cells in the context of muscular dystrophies

DMD is the most severe form of muscular dystrophies. It is the most common inherited muscle disease of childhood afflicting approximately 1 in 3500 young males [77]. It is characterized as a muscular disorder caused by mutations in the dystrophin gene located on the short arm of the X chromosome. The absence of, or defects in, dystrophin results in chronic inflammation, progressive muscle degeneration, and replacement of muscle with fibroadipose tissues [77]. DMD patients often lose independent ambulation by the time they reach 13 years of age and generally die of respiratory failure in their late teens or early twenties [78]. Myotonic dystrophy type 1 (DM1) and type 2 (DM2) represent the most frequent multisystemic muscular dystrophies in adulthood [79]. DM1 and DM2 are rare disorders caused by noncoding intragenic repeat tract expansions of CTG (*DMPK* gene) and CCTG (*CNBP1* gene), which are pathogenic above 50 or 75 units, respectively [80, 81]. DM patients have primarily affected skeletal musculature and display muscle weakness (myopathy), muscle wasting (atrophy), and myotonia as the most recognized signs [79, 81]. DM1 and DM2 are characterized as multisystem progressive disorders, with the most frequent causes of death being respiratory failure and heart conduction defects.

Comprehensive miRNA expression profiling has revealed that miRNA dysregulation is a common feature in DMD and DM muscles. Nevertheless, the specific role that this dysregulation exerts over dystrophic muscle precursor cell biology is poorly understood. In this sense, Alexander et al. showed that miR-486 is down-regulated in human DMD myoblast during myogenic differentiation as they are compared with wild type [50]. As we have mentioned before, this miR acts as a negative regulator of the PTEN/AKT signaling components and their downstream effector during skeletal muscle regeneration [50]. Lack of miR-486 PTEN/AKT signaling deregulation worsens myoblast differentiation and, consequently, could aggravate the DMD phenotype. Hence, modulation of the PTEN/AKT signaling pathway through miR-486 expression has the potential to be a therapy for treating DMD. Nevertheless, this hypothesis remains elusive. The same group has also showed that miR-199a is overexpressed in human DMD myoblast during myogenic differentiation as they are compared with wild type [65]. As we have mentioned before, miR-199a acts as a potential regulator of myogenesis through suppression of WNT signaling factors that act to balance myogenic cell proliferation and differentiation. Alexander et al. showed how muscle-specific overexpression of miR-199a transcript *in vivo* results in myofiber disruption and early lethality in zebrafish. However, in this work, the authors use a mylz2-promoter sequence to drive miR-199a-5p expression in skeletal muscle. This promoter is active specifically in zebrafish skeletal muscle fibers, excluding muscle stem cell progenitors [82], hence the effect of miR-199a overexpression in muscle precursor cells still remain unknown. Nevertheless, modulation of miR-199a also emerges with an important potential to be a therapy for treating DMD. In a more specific approach, de Arcangelis et al. showed that the expression level of miR-222 was 50% higher in SCs from dystrophic mdx muscles than in wild type cells. This leads to the decrease in β1-syntrophin expression by specifically binding to the 3′-UTR of β 1-syntrophin, a component of dystrophin-associated protein complex (DAPC), suggesting that the absence of β1-syntrophin could worsen the disease [83]. Nevertheless, the authors did not explore downstream effects mediated by miR-222 overexpression in SCs, hence its impact in muscle precursor cells still remains elusive.

To obtain primary dystrophic muscle precursors cell cultures, either SCs or their derived myoblasts, is an extreme difficult task to achieve since their pathological backgrounds prevent their proper expansion *in vitro*. Some groups have tried to partially solve this problem by obtaining myogenic cell lines from dystrophic patients derived from immortalized fibroblasts by using retroviral-mediated expression of murine MyoD under the control of the Tet-on inducible construct or by transduction of the TERT and inducible Myod genes [84, 85]. By using this approach, Fernandez-Costa et al. showed that, as happened in DM1 Drosophila model muscle cells, myogenic cell lines derived from DM1 patients showed a downregulation of miR-1, miR-7, and miR-10, demonstrating the conservation of miRNA dysregulation triggered by expanded CTG repeats between the Drosophila model and humans [85]. Although overexpression of some of their putative targets was validated by RT-qPCR, the mechanisms by which this downregulation induces in DM1-myoblast maturation still remains unknown. Similarly, Cappella et al. showed a significant miRNA29c downregulation in human DM1 myotubes [84]. Since miRNA29c targets ankyrin repeat and SOCS box containing 2 (Asb2), a subunit of a multimeric E3 ubiquitin-ligase complex that negatively regulates muscle fiber mass [84], miRNA29c downregulation in DM1 could affect total muscle mass and worsen disease progression. In agreement with Cappella et al., Wang et al. (2012) have demonstrated that the loss of miR-29 impairs myogenic differentiation in mdx myoblasts [86]. This impairment may be due to the control exercised by miR29 in fibrosis.

In this regard, we must stress that miR-29-family miRNAs display a crucial role in the regulation of extracellular matrix genes and in fibrosis [87]. The replacement of muscle with fibroadipose tissues is a major pathological hallmark of DMD and DM [77, 84]. The canonical TGF-β/Smad signaling pathway, a well-known pathway involved in fibrosis formation, appears to negatively regulate the expression of miR-29, thereby promoting the conversion of myoblasts in myofibroblasts [86, 88]. During this transdifferentiation, activated TGF-β signaling induces Smad3 translocation into nucleus where it binds to miR-29 promoter, resulting in MyoD dissociation as well as YY1/Ezh2 stabilization. This causes a loss of miR-29 expression and increased expression of collagens and Lims1, leading to the transdifferentiation of myoblasts into myofibroblasts. All together, these data suggest that miR-29 could be an important molecular target for treating fibrosis associated to DMD and DM phenotypes.

Beyond the mere description, the works presented in this section provide us with very valuable information that can help us find new therapeutic targets on which to focus the development of drugs that would help us to alleviate the effects of dystrophic pathologies. We will discuss this issue in the next section.

5.2 miRNA as therapeutic targets in DMD and DM

As we have previously illustrated, several miRNAs are significantly dysregulated in DMD and DM muscular dystrophies and are able to modify muscle cell behavior in this context. For those downregulated, miRNA replacement can be conducted to restore its function by introducing a miRNA mimic product. The miR mimic technology utilizes synthetic, modified oligonucleotides that can bind to the unique sequence of target genes (mRNAs) in a gene-specific manner and elicit posttranscriptional repressive effects as an endogenous miRNA does [89]. Alternatively, application of miR mimics targeting the disease-causing genes to prevent their upregulation may be an efficient maneuver to tackle the problem [89]. For those miRNAs upregulated, inhibition can be conducted by using antimiR products.

Different types of antimiR products exist based on their mechanism of action. As happens for the miRNA mimic product, antimiRs comprise numerous classes of chemically modified oligonucleotides and nucleic acid analogs like locked nucleic acids (LNAs), 2′-O-methyl (2′-O-Me) oligos, 2′-O-methoxyethyl (2′-O-MOE) oligos, antagomiRs, peptide nucleic acids (PNAs), and phosphorodiamidate morpholinos (PMOs) [90]. These chemical modifications are implemented to provide resistance to cellular nucleases and to increase affinity toward complementary miRNA sequences [91, 92]. In addition, some antimiRs have flanking sequences or are connected to lipids through the use of linkers [93]. All the molecules that we have mentioned so far induce transient effects either because they are diluted by successive cell divisions or because they are metabolized in the cytoplasm [93]. To achieve long-term suppression of a specific miRNA, specialized plasmid and virus vectors carrying expression units for these inhibitory RNA molecules have also been developed [94]. In this regard, as an alternative to chemically modified antisense oligonucleotides, Ebert et al. developed miRNA inhibitors that can be expressed in cells as RNAs produced from transgenes [95]. Termed "miRNA sponges," these competitive inhibitors are transcripts expressed from strong promoters, containing multiple, tandem binding sites to an miRNA of interest. When vectors encoding these sponges are transfected into cultured cells, sponges derepress miRNA targets at least as strongly as chemically modified antisense oligonucleotides [95].

Muscular dystrophy	Molecular approach	Mimic/target miRNA	References
Duchenne muscular dystrophy	miRNA mimic/antimiR	miR-21	[97, 98]
	miRNA mimic	miR-29	[86, 97, 99]
	miRNA sponge	miR-31	[100]
	miRNA mimic/antimiR	miR-34c	[101]
	miRNA mimic/antimiR	miR-188	[102]
	miRNA sponge	miR-206	[103]
	miRNA mimic	miR-431	[104]
	miRNA mimic/antimiR	miR-675	[98]
	miRNA mimic/antimiR	miR-708	[101]
	miRNA mimic	miR-10	[85]
	miRNA sponge	miR-277	[105]
Myotonic dystrophy	miRNA sponge	miR-304	[105]
	antimiR	miR-23b	[106]
	antimiR	miR-218	[106]
	miRNA mimic	miR-1	[107, 108]
	miRNA mimic	miR-206	[107, 109]
	miRNA mimic	miR-148a	[107]
	miRNA mimic	miR-214	[107]
	miRNA mimic	miR-15b	[107]
	miRNA mimic	miR-16	[107]
	miRNA mimic	miR-30	[110]

Table 2.
miRs' therapeutic assays in animal models.

These miRNA sponge vectors inhibit miRNA function efficiently but for no longer than 1 month [96]. This problem has been partially solved by the development of "tough decoy RNAs" technology [93, 96]. Tough decoy inhibitor is a 60 base pair long hairpin-shaped inhibitor with a large internal bulge containing two miRNA recognition sites [93, 96]. Through plasmid- or lentivirus-based vectors, these molecules are efficiently exportable to the cytoplasm, where they target the highly potent miRNA inhibitory system which persists for well over 1 month [93, 96]. In the field of muscular dystrophies, many of these approaches have been tested *in vitro* and *in vivo* with animal models (**Table 2**). However, doubts related to the safety and efficiency of delivery still discourage the use of these molecules in humans.

6. Conclusions and perspectives

At present, a critical point for the development of effective strategies for treating muscle disorders is optimizing approaches to target muscle stem cells in order to increase the ability to regenerate lost tissue. In the context of muscle regeneration, emerging scientific evidence supports that *miRNAs* play a critical role in skeletal muscle, as they are required for the development and differentiation of this tissue. In addition, deregulation of *miRNAs* in muscle degenerative diseases suggests that gene-based therapies of *miRNAs* can be effective in treating muscle-related disorders. In this sense, restoration of non-pathological level of miRs expression would help to ameliorate these pathologies. Although many *in vitro* approaches have been accomplished in this regard, *in vivo* strategies remain poorly explored since the main shortcoming of the field lies in the ineffective delivery of either mimics or antimiR molecules. These molecules must overcome numerous roadblocks as canonical physiological pharmacokinetic and cellular uptake barriers as well as noncanonical barriers, such as intracellular miRNA localization and trafficking, off-target toxicities, and other intrinsic limitations. Improvement in this task will be the upcoming challenge for the next years by looking for strategies that allow us to aim these molecules in a specific fashion to muscle progenitor cells, thus minimizing the off-target effects of non-muscle tissues.

Conflicts of interest

The authors declare no conflict of interest.

Author contributions

Francisco Hernandez-Torres and Amelia Aranega conceived of the structure and content. Francisco Hernandez-Torres wrote the first draft document. Francisco Hernandez-Torres, Lara Rodriguez-Outeiriño, and Lidia Matias-Valiente designed and produced the figures and tables. Estefania Lozano-Velasco and Diego Franco critically revised the manuscript for intellectual content. All authors provided content and writing feedback and reviewed the final manuscript. Amelia Aranega corrected, edited, and approved the final version of the document to be published.

Funding

This work is supported by Duchenne Parent Project-DPP2019.

Author details

Francisco Hernandez-Torres[1,2,3], Lara Rodriguez-Outeiriño[1,2], Lidia Matias-Valiente[1,2], Estefania Lozano-Velasco[1,2], Diego Franco[1,2] and Amelia Aranega[1,2]*

1 Department of Experimental Biology, University of Jaen, Jaen, Spain

2 Medina Foundation, Technology Park of Health Sciences, Granada, Spain

3 Department of Biochemistry and Molecular Biology III and Immunology, University of Granada, Granada, Spain

*Address all correspondence to: aaranega@ujaen.es

References

[1] Janssen I, Heymsfield SB, Wang ZM, Ross R. Skeletal muscle mass and distribution in 468 men and women aged 18-88 yr. Journal of Applied Physiology. 2000;**89**:81-88. DOI: 10.1152/jappl.2000.89.1.81

[2] Almada AE, Wagers AJ. Molecular circuitry of stem cell fate in skeletal muscle regeneration, ageing and disease. Nature Reviews. Molecular Cell Biology. 2016;**17**:267-279. DOI: 10.1038/nrm.2016.7

[3] Mauro A. Satellite cell of skeletal muscle fibers. The Journal of Biophysical and Biochemical Cytology. 1961;**9**:493-495. DOI: 10.1083/jcb.9.2.493

[4] Armand O, Boutineau AM, Mauger A, Pautou MP, Kieny M. Origin of satellite cells in avian skeletal muscles. Archives d'Anatomie Microscopique et de Morphologie Expérimentale. 1983;**72**:163-181

[5] Relaix F, Rocancourt D, Mansouri A, Buckingham M. A Pax3/Pax7-dependent population of skeletal muscle progenitor cells. Nature. 2005;**435**: 948-953. DOI: 10.1038/nature03594

[6] Schienda J, Engleka KA, Jun S, Hansen MS, Epstein JA, Tabin CJ, et al. Somitic origin of limb muscle satellite and side population cells. Proceedings of the National Academy of Sciences of the United States of America. 2006;**103**:945-950. DOI: 10.1073/pnas.0510164103

[7] Harel I, Nathan E, Tirosh-Finkel L, Zigdon H, Guimarães-Camboa N, Evans SM, et al. Distinct origins and genetic programs of head muscle satellite cells. Developmental Cell. 2009;**16**:822-832. DOI: 10.1016/j.devcel.2009.05.007

[8] Zanou N, Gailly P. Skeletal muscle hypertrophy and regeneration: Interplay between the myogenic regulatory factors (MRFs) and insulin-like growth factors (IGFs) pathways. Cellular and Molecular Life Sciences. 2013;**70**:4117-4130. DOI: 10.1007/s00018-013-1330-4

[9] Lee Y, Kim M, Han J, Yeom KH, Lee S, Baek SH, et al. MicroRNA genes are transcribed by RNA polymerase II. The EMBO Journal. 2004;**23**:4051-4060. DOI: 10.1038/sj.emboj.7600385

[10] Godnic I, Zorc M, Jevsinek Skok D, Calin GA, Horvat S, Dovc P, et al. Genome-wide and species-wide In silico screening for intragenic MicroRNAs in human, mouse and chicken. PLoS One. 2013;**8**:e65165. DOI: 10.1371/journal.pone.0065165

[11] Lee Y, Ahn C, Han J, Choi H, Kim J, Yim J, et al. The nuclear RNase III Drosha initiates microRNA processing. Nature. 2003;**425**:415-419. DOI: 10.1038/nature01957

[12] Wang X, Xu X, Ma Z, Huo Y, Xiao Z, Li Y, et al. Dynamic mechanisms for pre-miRNA binding and export by Exportin-5. RNA. 2011;**17**:1511-1528. DOI: 10.1261/rna.2732611

[13] Ketting RF, Fischer SEJ, Bernstein E, Sijen T, Hannon GJ, Plasterk RHA. Dicer functions in RNA interference and in synthesis of small RNA involved in developmental timing in *C. elegans*. Genes & Development. 2001;**15**: 2654-2659. DOI: 10.1101/gad.927801

[14] MacRae IJ, Zhou K, Li F, Repic A, Brooks AN, Cande WZ, et al. Structural basis for double-stranded RNA processing by Dicer. Science. 2006;**311**:195-198. DOI: 10.1126/science.1121638

[15] Pasquinelli AE. MicroRNAs and their targets: Recognition, regulation and an emerging reciprocal relationship. Nature Reviews. Genetics. 2012;**13**: 271-282. DOI: 10.1038/nrg3162

[16] Abdelfattah AM, Park C, Choi MY. Update on non-canonical microRNAs. Biomolecular Concepts. 2014;**5**:275-287. DOI: 10.1515/bmc-2014-0012

[17] Kim YK, Kim VN. Processing of intronic microRNAs. The EMBO Journal. 2007;**26**:775-783. DOI: 10.1038/sj.emboj.7601512

[18] Rearick D, Prakash A, McSweeny A, Shepard SS, Fedorova L, Fedorov A. Critical association of ncRNA with introns. Nucleic Acids Research. 2011;**39**:2357-2366. DOI: 10.1093/nar/gkq1080

[19] Paneru BD, Al-Tobasei R, Kenney B, Leeds TD, Salem M. RNA-seq reveals MicroRNA expression signature and genetic polymorphism associated with growth and muscle quality traits in rainbow trout. Scientific Reports. 2017;**7**:1-15. DOI: 10.1038/s41598-017-09515-4

[20] Castel D, Baghdadi MB, Mella S, Gayraud-Morel B, Marty V, Cavaillé J, et al. Small-RNA sequencing identifies dynamic microRNA deregulation during skeletal muscle lineage progression. Scientific Reports. 2018;**8**:1-13. DOI: 10.1038/s41598-018-21991-w

[21] Coenen-Stass AML, Sork H, Gatto S, Godfrey C, Bhomra A, Krjutškov K, et al. Comprehensive RNA-sequencing analysis in serum and muscle reveals novel Small RNA signatures with biomarker potential for DMD. Molecular Therapy--Nucleic Acids. 2018;**13**:1-15. DOI: 10.1016/j.omtn.2018.08.005

[22] Zhao Y, Ransom JF, Li A, Vedantham V, von Drehle M, Muth AN, et al. Dysregulation of Cardiogenesis, cardiac conduction, and cell cycle in mice lacking miRNA-1-2. Cell. 2007;**129**:303-317. DOI: 10.1016/j.cell.2007.03.030

[23] Liu N, Bezprozvannaya S, Williams AH, Qi X, Richardson JA, Bassel-Duby R, et al. microRNA-133a regulates cardiomyocyte proliferation and suppresses smooth muscle gene expression in the heart. Genes & Development. 2008;**22**:3242-3254. DOI: 10.1101/gad.1738708

[24] Williams AH, Valdez G, Moresi V, Qi X, McAnally J, Elliott JL, et al. MicroRNA-206 delays ALS progression and promotes regeneration of neuromuscular synapses in mice. Science. 2009;**326**:1549-1554. DOI: 10.1126/science.1181046

[25] Van Rooij E, Sutherland LB, Qi X, Richardson JA, Hill J, Olson EN. Control of stress-dependent cardiac growth and gene expression by a microRNA. Science. 2007;**316**:575-579. DOI: 10.1126/science.1139089

[26] Callis TE, Pandya K, Hee YS, Tang RH, Tatsuguchi M, Huang ZP, et al. MicroRNA-208a is a regulator of cardiac hypertrophy and conduction in mice. The Journal of Clinical Investigation. 2009;**119**:2772-2786. DOI: 10.1172/JCI36154

[27] van Rooij E, Quiat D, Johnson BA, Sutherland LB, Qi X, Richardson JA, et al. A family of microRNAs encoded by myosin genes governs myosin expression and muscle performance. Developmental Cell. 2009;**17**:662-673. DOI: 10.1016/j.devcel.2009.10.013

[28] Small EM, O'Rourke JR, Moresi V, Sutherland LB, McAnally J, Gerard RD, et al. Regulation of PI3-kinase/Akt signaling by muscle-enriched microRNA-486. Proceedings of the National Academy of Sciences of the United States of America. 2010;**107**:4218-4223. DOI: 10.1073/pnas.1000300107

[29] McCarthy JJ. The myomiR network in skeletal muscle plasticity. Exercise and Sport Sciences Reviews. 2011;**39**:150-154. DOI: 10.1097/JES.0b013e31821c01e1

[30] Cheung TH, Quach NL, Charville GW, Liu L, Park L, Edalati A, et al. Maintenance of muscle stem-cell quiescence by microRNA-489. Nature. 2012;**482**:524-528. DOI: 10.1038/nature10834

[31] Crist CG, Montarras D, Buckingham M. Muscle satellite cells are primed for myogenesis but maintain quiescence with sequestration of Myf5 mRNA targeted by microRNA-31 in mRNP granules. Cell Stem Cell. 2012;**11**:118-126. DOI: 10.1016/j.stem.2012.03.011

[32] Baghdadi MB, Firmino J, Soni K, Evano B, Di Girolamo D, Mourikis P, et al. Notch-induced miR-708 antagonizes satellite cell migration and maintains quiescence. Cell Stem Cell. 2018;**23**:859-868.e5. DOI: 10.1016/j.stem.2018.09.017

[33] Chen JF, Mandel EM, Thomson JM, Wu Q, Callis TE, Hammond SM, et al. The role of microRNA-1 and microRNA-133 in skeletal muscle proliferation and differentiation. Nature Genetics. 2006;**38**:228-233. DOI: 10.1038/ng1725

[34] Cai R, Qimuge N, Ma M, Wang Y, Tang G, Zhang Q, et al. MicroRNA-664-5p promotes myoblast proliferation and inhibits myoblast differentiation by targeting serum response factor and Wnt1. The Journal of Biological Chemistry. 2018;**293**:19177-19190. DOI: 10.1074/jbc.RA118.003198

[35] Huang Z, Chen X, Yu B, He J, Chen D. MicroRNA-27a promotes myoblast proliferation by targeting myostatin. Biochemical and Biophysical Research Communications. 2012;**423**:265-269. DOI: 10.1016/j.bbrc.2012.05.106

[36] Qiu H, Liu N, Luo L, Zhong J, Tang Z, Kang K, et al. MicroRNA-17-92 regulates myoblast proliferation and differentiation by targeting the ENH1/Id1 signaling axis. Cell Death and Differentiation. 2016;**23**:1658-1669. DOI: 10.1038/cdd.2016.56

[37] Wei W, Zhang WY, Bai JB, Zhang HX, Zhao YY, Li XY, et al. The NF-κB-modulated microRNAs miR-195 and miR-497 inhibit myoblast proliferation by targeting Igf1r, Insr and cyclin genes. Journal of Cell Science. 2016;**129**:39-50. DOI: 10.1242/jcs.174235

[38] Wang J, Tan J, Qi Q, Yang L, Wang Y, Zhang C, et al. MiR-487b-3p suppresses the proliferation and differentiation of myoblasts by targeting IRS1 in skeletal muscle myogenesis. International Journal of Biological Sciences. 2018;**14**:760-774. DOI: 10.7150/ijbs.25052

[39] Jia X, Ouyang H, Abdalla BA, Xu H, Nie Q, Zhang X. miR-16 controls myoblast proliferation and apoptosis through directly suppressing Bcl2 and FOXO1 activities. Biochimica et Biophysica Acta, Gene Regulatory Mechanisms. 2017;**1860**:674-684. DOI: 10.1016/j.bbagrm.2017.02.010

[40] Zhang D, Li X, Chen C, Li Y, Zhao L, Jing Y, et al. Attenuation of p38-mediated miR-1/133 expression facilitates myoblast proliferation during the early stage of muscle regeneration. PLoS One. 2012;**7**:e41478 (Electronic version). DOI: 10.1371/journal.pone.0041478

[41] Lozano-Velasco E, Vallejo D, Esteban FJ, Doherty C, Hernández-Torres F, Franco D, et al. A Pitx2 -MicroRNA pathway modulates cell proliferation in myoblasts and skeletal-muscle satellite cells and promotes their commitment to a myogenic cell fate. Molecular and Cellular Biology. 2015;**35**:2892-2909. DOI: 10.1128/mcb.00536-15

[42] Chen JF, Tao Y, Li J, Deng Z, Yan Z, Xiao X, et al. microRNA-1 and microRNA-206 regulate skeletal

muscle satellite cell proliferation and differentiation by repressing Pax7. The Journal of Cell Biology. 2010;**190**:867-879. DOI: 10.1083/jcb.200911036

[43] Cacchiarelli D, Martone J, Girardi E, Cesana M, Incitti T, Morlando M, et al. Cell metabolism article microRNAs involved in molecular circuitries relevant for the Duchenne muscular dystrophy pathogenesis are controlled by the dystrophin/nNOS pathway. Cell Metabolism. 2010;**12**:341-351. DOI: 10.1016/j.cmet.2010.07.008

[44] Liu N, Williams AH, Maxeiner JM, Bezprozvannaya S, Shelton JM, Richardson JA, et al. MicroRNA-206 promotes skeletal muscle regeneration and delays progression of Duchenne muscular dystrophy in mice. The Journal of Clinical Investigation. 2012;**122**:2054-2065. DOI: 10.1172/JCI62656

[45] Hak KK, Yong SL, Sivaprasad U, Malhotra A, Dutta A. Muscle-specific microRNA miR-206 promotes muscle differentiation. The Journal of Cell Biology. 2006;**174**:677-687. DOI: 10.1083/jcb.200603008

[46] Anderson C, Catoe H, Werner R. MIR-206 regulates connexin43 expression during skeletal muscle development. Nucleic Acids Research. 2006;**34**:5863-5871. DOI: 10.1093/nar/gkl743

[47] Dey BK, Gagan J, Dutta A. miR-206 and -486 induce myoblast differentiation by downregulating Pax7. Molecular and Cellular Biology. 2011;**31**:203-214. DOI: 10.1128/mcb.01009-10

[48] Miyauchi H, Minamino T, Tateno K, Kunieda T, Toko H, Komuro I. Akt negatively regulates the in vitro lifespan of human endothelial cells via a p53/p21-dependent pathway. The EMBO Journal. 2004;**23**:212-220. DOI: 10.1038/sj.emboj.7600045

[49] Lees SJ, Childs TE, Booth FW. Age-dependent FOXO regulation of p27Kip1 expression via a conserved binding motif in rat muscle precursor cells. American Journal of Physiology. Cell Physiology. 2008;**295**:C1238-C1246. DOI: 10.1152/ajpcell.00349.2008

[50] Alexander MS, Casar JC, Motohashi N, Myers JA, Eisenberg I, Gonzalez RT, et al. Regulation of DMD pathology by an ankyrin-encoded miRNA. Skeletal Muscle. 2011;**1**:27. DOI: 10.1186/2044-5040-1-27

[51] Feng Y, Niu LL, Wei W, Zhang WY, Li XY, Cao JH, et al. A feedback circuit between miR-133 and the ERK1/2 pathway involving an exquisite mechanism for regulating myoblast proliferation and differentiation. Cell Death & Disease. 2013;**4**:e934. DOI: 10.1038/cddis.2013.462

[52] Zhou L, Wang L, Lu L, Jiang P, Sun H, Wang H. A novel target of microRNA-29, Ring1 and YY1-binding protein (Rybp), negatively regulates skeletal myogenesis. The Journal of Biological Chemistry. 2012;**287**:25255-25265. DOI: 10.1074/jbc.M112.357053

[53] Winbanks CE, Wang B, Beyer C, Koh P, White L, Kantharidis P, et al. TGF-β regulates miR-206 and miR-29 to control myogenic differentiation through regulation of HDAC4. The Journal of Biological Chemistry. 2011;**286**:13805-13814. DOI: 10.1074/jbc.M110.192625

[54] Wei W, He HB, Zhang WY, Zhang HX, Bai JB, Liu HZ, et al. MiR-29 targets Akt3 to reduce proliferation and facilitate differentiation of myoblasts in skeletal muscle development. Cell Death & Disease. 2013;**4**:e668. DOI: 10.1038/cddis.2013.184

[55] Chung FW, Tellam RL. MicroRNA-26a targets the histone methyltransferase enhancer of zeste homolog 2 during myogenesis. The Journal of Biological Chemistry. 2008;**283**:9836-9843. DOI: 10.1074/jbc.M709614200

[56] Dey BK, Gagan J, Yan Z, Dutta A. miR-26a is required for skeletal muscle differentiation and regeneration in mice. Genes & Development. 2012;**26**:2180-2191. DOI: 10.1101/gad.198085.112

[57] Juan AH, Kumar RM, Marx JG, Young RA, Sartorelli V. Mir-214-dependent regulation of the polycomb protein Ezh2 in skeletal muscle and embryonic stem cells. Molecular Cell. 2009;**36**:61-74. DOI: 10.1016/j.molcel.2009.08.008

[58] Liu J, Luo XJ, Xiong AW, Zeng-di Z, Yue S, Zhu MS, et al. MicroRNA-214 promotes myogenic differentiation by facilitating exit from mitosis via down-regulation of proto-oncogene N-ras. The Journal of Biological Chemistry. 2010;**285**:26599-26607. DOI: 10.1074/jbc.M110.115824

[59] Naguibneva I, Ameyar-Zazoua M, Polesskaya A, Ait-Si-Ali S, Groisman R, Souidi M, et al. The microRNA miR-181 targets the homeobox protein Hox-A11 during mammalian myoblast differentiation. Nature Cell Biology. 2006;**8**:278-284. DOI: 10.1038/ncb1373

[60] Gagan J, Dey BK, Layer R, Yan Z, Dutta A. MicroRNA-378 targets the myogenic repressor MyoR during myoblast differentiation. The Journal of Biological Chemistry. 2011;**286**:19431-19438. DOI: 10.1074/jbc.M111.219006

[61] Wang Z, Ouyang H, Chen X, Yu J, Abdalla BA, Chen B, et al. Gga-miR-205a affecting myoblast proliferation and differentiation by targeting CDH11. Frontiers in Genetics. 2018;**9**:414. DOI: 10.3389/fgene.2018.00414

[62] Dey BK, Pfeifer K, Dutta A. The H19 long noncoding RNA gives rise to microRNAs miR-675-3p and miR-675-5p to promote skeletal muscle differentiation and regeneration. Genes & Development. 2014;**28**:491-501. DOI: 10.1101/gad.234419.113

[63] Kong D, He M, Yang L, Zhou R, Yan YQ, Liang Y, et al. MiR-17 and miR-19 cooperatively promote skeletal muscle cell differentiation. Cellular and Molecular Life Sciences. 2019;**76**:5041-5054. DOI: 10.1007/s00018-019-03165-7

[64] Wang Z, Li A, Chen N. MiR-34b-5p mediates the proliferation and differentiation of myoblasts by targeting IGFBP2. Cell. 2019;**8**:360. DOI: 10.3390/cells8040360

[65] Alexander MS, Kawahara G, Motohashi N, Casar JC, Eisenberg I, Myers JA, et al. MicroRNA-199a is induced in dystrophic muscle and affects WNT signaling, cell proliferation, and myogenic differentiation. Cell Death and Differentiation. 2013;**20**:1194-1208. DOI: 10.1038/cdd.2013.62

[66] Seok HY, Tatsuguchi M, Callis TE, He A, Pu WT, Wang DZ. miR-155 inhibits expression of the MEF2A protein to repress skeletal muscle differentiation. The Journal of Biological Chemistry. 2011;**286**:35339-35346. DOI: 10.1074/jbc.M111.273276

[67] Du J, Zhang P, Zhao X, He J, Xu Y, Zou Q, et al. MicroRNA-351-5p mediates skeletal myogenesis by directly targeting lactamase-β and is regulated by lnc-mg. The FASEB Journal. 2019;**33**:1911-1926. DOI: 10.1096/fj.201701394RRR

[68] Wang L, Chen X, Zheng Y, Li F, Lu Z, Chen C, et al. MiR-23a inhibits myogenic differentiation through down regulation of fast myosin heavy chain isoforms. Experimental Cell Research. 2012;**318**:2324-2334. DOI: 10.1016/j.yexcr.2012.06.018

[69] Yuan Y, Shi XE, Liu YG, Yang GS. FoxO1 regulates muscle fiber-type specification and inhibits calcineurin signaling during C2C12 myoblast differentiation. Molecular and Cellular

Biochemistry. 2011;**348**:77-87. DOI: 10.1007/s11010-010-0640-1

[70] Parakati R, DiMario JX. Repression of myoblast proliferation and fibroblast growth factor receptor 1 promoter activity by KLF10 protein. The Journal of Biological Chemistry. 2013;**288**:13876-13884. DOI: 10.1074/jbc.M113.457648

[71] Lu J, McKinsey TA, Zhang CL, Olson EN. Regulation of skeletal myogenesis by association of the MEF2 transcription factor with class II histone deacetylases. Molecular Cell. 2000;**6**:233-244. DOI: 10.1016/S1097-2765(00)00025-3

[72] Wang H, Garzon R, Sun H, Ladner KJ, Singh R, Dahlman J, et al. NF-κB-YY1-miR-29 regulatory circuitry in skeletal myogenesis and rhabdomyosarcoma. Cancer Cell. 2008;**14**:369-381. DOI: 10.1016/j.ccr.2008.10.006

[73] Buckingham M, Rigby PWJ. Gene regulatory networks and transcriptional mechanisms that control myogenesis. Developmental Cell. 2014;**28**:225-238. DOI: 10.1016/j.devcel.2013.12.020

[74] Zhu M, Liu J, Xiao J, Yang L, Cai M, Shen H, et al. Lnc-mg is a long non-coding RNA that promotes myogenesis. Nature Communications. 2017;**8**:14718. DOI: 10.1038/ncomms14718

[75] Kirby TJ, Chaillou T, McCarthy JJ. The role of microRNAs in skeletal muscle health and disease. Frontiers in Bioscience - Landmark. 2015;**20**:37-77. DOI: 10.2741/4298

[76] Emery AEH. The muscular dystrophies. Lancet, Elsevier Limited. 2002;**359**:687-695. DOI: 10.1016/S0140-6736(02)07815-7

[77] Mercuri E, Muntoni F. Muscular dystrophies. Lancet. 2013;**381**:845-860. DOI: 10.1016/S0140-6736(12)61897-2

[78] Mah JK, Korngut L, Dykeman J, Day L, Pringsheim T, Jette N. A systematic review and meta-analysis on the epidemiology of Duchenne and Becker muscular dystrophy. Neuromuscular Disorders. 2014;**24**:482-491. DOI: 10.1016/j.nmd.2014.03.008

[79] Wenninger S, Montagnese F, Schoser B. Core clinical phenotypes in myotonic dystrophies. Frontiers in Neurology. 2018;**9**:303. DOI: 10.3389/fneur.2018.00303

[80] Thornton CA. Myotonic dystrophy. Neurologic Clinics. 2014;**32**:705-719. DOI: 10.1016/j.ncl.2014.04.011

[81] Castel AL, Overby SJ, Artero R. MicroRNA-based therapeutic perspectives in myotonic dystrophy. International Journal of Molecular Sciences. 2019;**20**. DOI: 10.3390/ijms20225600

[82] Ju B, Chong SW, He J, Wang X, Xu Y, Wan H, et al. Recapitulation of fast skeletal muscle development in zebrafish by transgenic expression of GFP under the mylz2 promoter. Developmental Dynamics. 2003;**227**:14-26. DOI: 10.1002/dvdy.10273

[83] de Arcangelis V, Serra F, Cogoni C, Vivarelli E, Monaco L, Naro F. β1-syntrophin modulation by miR-222 in mdx mice. PLOS One. 2010;**5**. DOI: 10.1371/journal.pone.0012098

[84] Cappella M, Perfetti A, Cardinali B, Garcia-Manteiga JM, Carrara M, Provenzano C, et al. High-throughput analysis of the RNA-induced silencing complex in myotonic dystrophy type 1 patients identifies the dysregulation of miR-29c and its target ASB2. Cell Death & Disease. 2018;**9**:1-11. DOI: 10.1038/s41419-018-0769-5

[85] Fernandez-Costa JM, Garcia-Lopez A, Zuñiga S, Fernandez-Pedrosa V, Felipo-Benavent A, Mata M, et al. Expanded CTG repeats trigger

miRNA alterations in Drosophila that are conserved in myotonic dystrophy type 1 patients. Human Molecular Genetics. 2013;**22**:704-716. DOI: 10.1093/hmg/dds478

[86] Wang L, Zhou L, Jiang P, Lu L, Chen X, Lan H, et al. Loss of miR-29 in myoblasts contributes to dystrophic muscle pathogenesis. Molecular Therapy. 2012;**20**:1222-1233. DOI: 10.1038/mt.2012.35

[87] Deng Z, He Y, Yang X, Shi H, Shi A, Lu L, et al. MicroRNA-29: A crucial player in fibrotic disease. Molecular Diagnosis & Therapy. 2017;**21**:285-294. DOI: 10.1007/s40291-016-0253-9

[88] Zhou L, Wang L, Lu L, Jiang P, Sun H, Wang H. Inhibition of miR-29 by TGF-beta-Smad3 signaling through dual mechanisms promotes transdifferentiation of mouse myoblasts into myofibroblasts. PLOS One. 2012;**7**:e33766. DOI: 10.1371/journal.pone.0033766

[89] Wang Z. The guideline of the design and validation of miRNA mimics. Methods in Molecular Biology. 2011;**676**:211-223. DOI: 10.1007/978-1-60761-863-8_15

[90] Cheng CJ, Saltzman WM, Slack FJ. Canonical and non-canonical barriers facing antimiR cancer therapeutics. Current Medicinal Chemistry. 2013;**20**:3582-3593. DOI: 10.2174/0929867311320290004

[91] Davis S, Lollo B, Freier S, Esau C. Improved targeting of miRNA with antisense oligonucleotides. Nucleic Acids Research. 2006;**34**:2294-2304. DOI: 10.1093/nar/gkl183

[92] Ørom UA, Kauppinen S, Lund AH. LNA-modified oligonucleotides mediate specific inhibition of microRNA function. Gene. 2006;**372**:137-141. DOI: 10.1016/j.gene.2005.12.031

[93] Haraguchi T, Nakano H, Tagawa T, Ohki T, Ueno Y, Yoshida T, et al. A potent 2'-O-methylated RNA-based microRNA inhibitor with unique secondary structures. Nucleic Acids Research. 2012;**40**:e58. DOI: 10.1093/nar/gkr1317

[94] Scherr M, Venturini L, Battmer K, Schaller-Schoenitz M, Schaefer D, Dallmann I, et al. Lentivirus-mediated antagomir expression for specific inhibition of miRNA function. Nucleic Acids Research. 2007;**35**:e149. DOI: 10.1093/nar/gkm971

[95] Ebert MS, Neilson JR, Sharp PA. MicroRNA sponges: Competitive inhibitors of small RNAs in mammalian cells. Nature Methods. 2007;**4**:721-726. DOI: 10.1038/nmeth1079

[96] Haraguchi T, Ozaki Y, Iba H. Vectors expressing efficient RNA decoys achieve the long-term suppression of specific microRNA activity in mammalian cells. Nucleic Acids Research. 2009;**37**:43. DOI: 10.1093/nar/gkp040

[97] Zanotti S, Gibertini S, Curcio M, Savadori P, Pasanisi B, Morandi L, et al. Opposing roles of miR-21 and miR-29 in the progression of fibrosis in Duchenne muscular dystrophy. Biochimica et Biophysica Acta, Molecular Basis of Disease. 1852;**2015**:1451-1464. DOI: 10.1016/j.bbadis.2015.04.013

[98] Morgoulis D, Berenstein P, Cazacu S, Kazimirsky G, Dori A, Barnea ER, et al. sPIF promotes myoblast differentiation and utrophin expression while inhibiting fibrosis in Duchenne muscular dystrophy via the H19/miR-675/let-7 and miR-21 pathways. Cell Death & Disease. 2019;**10**:1-10. DOI: 10.1038/s41419-019-1307-9

[99] Heller KN, Mendell JT, Mendell JR, Rodino-Klapac LR. MicroRNA-29 overexpression by adeno-associated

virus suppresses fibrosis and restores muscle function in combination with micro-dystrophin. JCI Insight. 2017;**2**. DOI: 10.1172/jci.insight.93309

[100] Cacchiarelli D, Incitti T, Martone J, Cesana M, Cazzella V, Santini T, et al. MiR-31 modulates dystrophin expression: New implications for Duchenne muscular dystrophy therapy. EMBO Reports. 2011;**12**:136-141. DOI: 10.1038/embor.2010.208

[101] Guilbaud M, Gentil C, Peccate C, Gargaun E, Holtzmann I, Gruszczynski C, et al. miR-708-5p and miR-34c-5p are involved in nNOS regulation in dystrophic context. Skeletal Muscle. 2018;**8**:15. DOI: 10.1186/s13395-018-0161-2

[102] Shibasaki H, Imamura M, Arima S, Tanihata J, Kuraoka M, Matsuzaka Y, et al. Characterization of a novel microRNA, miR-188, elevated in serum of muscular dystrophy dog model. PLOS One. 2019;**14**. DOI: 10.1371/journal.pone.0211597

[103] Bulaklak K, Xiao B, Qiao C, Li J, Patel T, Jin Q, et al. MicroRNA-206 downregulation improves therapeutic gene expression and motor function in mdx mice. Molecular Therapy--Nucleic Acids. 2018;**12**:283-293. DOI: 10.1016/j.omtn.2018.05.011

[104] Wu R, Li H, Zhai L, Zou X, Meng J, Zhong R, et al. MicroRNA-431 accelerates muscle regeneration and ameliorates muscular dystrophy by targeting Pax7 in mice. Nature Communications. 2015;**6**:. DOI: 10.1038/ncomms8713

[105] Cerro-Herreros E, Fernandez-Costa JM, Sabater-Arcis M, Llamusi B, Artero R. Derepressing muscleblind expression by miRNA sponges ameliorates myotonic dystrophy-like phenotypes in Drosophila. Scientific Reports. 2016;**6**:1-13. DOI: 10.1038/srep36230

[106] Cerro-Herreros E, Sabater-Arcis M, Fernandez-Costa JM, Moreno N, Perez-Alonso M, Llamusi B, et al. MiR-23b and miR-218 silencing increase Muscleblind-like expression and alleviate myotonic dystrophy phenotypes in mammalian models. Nature Communications. 2018;**9**:1-13. DOI: 10.1038/s41467-018-04892-4

[107] Koscianska E, Witkos TM, Kozlowska E, Wojciechowska M, Krzyzosiak WJ. Cooperation meets competition in microRNA-mediated DMPK transcript regulation. Nucleic Acids Research. 2015;**43**(19):9500-9518. DOI: 10.1093/nar/gkv849

[108] Rau F, Freyermuth F, Fugier C, Villemin JP, Fischer MC, Jost B, et al. Misregulation of miR-1 processing is associated with heart defects in myotonic dystrophy. Nature Structural & Molecular Biology. 2011;**18**:840-845. DOI: 10.1038/nsmb.2067

[109] Dong W, Chen X, Wang M, Zheng Z, Zhang X, Xiao Q, et al. Mir-206 partially rescues myogenesis deficiency by inhibiting CUGBP1 accumulation in the cell models of myotonic dystrophy. Neurological Research. 2019;**41**:9-18. DOI: 10.1080/01616412.2018.1493963

[110] Zhang BW, Cai HF, Wei XF, Sun JJ, Lan XY, Lei CZ, et al. mir-30-5p regulates muscle differentiation and alternative splicing of muscle-related genes by targeting MBNL. International Journal of Molecular Sciences. 2016;**17**(2):182. DOI: 10.3390/ijms17020182

Chapter 4

Role of Growth Factors and Apoptosis Proteins in Cognitive Disorder Development in Patients with Duchenne Muscular Dystrophy

Mariia Georgievna Sokolova
and Ekaterina Valentinovna Lopatina

Abstract

Duchenne muscular dystrophy (DMD) is a progressive neuromuscular disease; it occurs due to a mutation in the dystrophin protein gene; as a result, the protein is not synthesized and muscle tissue dies. On the one hand, we can say that this disease has been sufficiently studied; however, it is still incurable, and there are a number of issues remaining unclear in terms of the development of progressive dementia as a symptom in 30% of patients with Duchenne muscular dystrophy. We conducted a study at the intersection of molecular genetic, neurological, and enzyme-linked immunosorbent patients' blood tests and experiments in organotypic culture, which allowed us to determine important points in the development of cognitive disorders in patients with Duchenne muscular dystrophy and identify a significant effect of growth factor concentration in patients. The chapter will present data on neurotrophic regulation in patients with Duchenne muscular dystrophy (by the best-studied neurotrophins), demonstrate special aspects of neuron-myocyte interaction, and broaden the understanding of the role of apoptosis and synthase proteins in the development of this disease. We would like to highlight the importance of prognostic criteria for the development of cognitive impairment and possible therapeutic measures to prevent progressive dementia

Keywords: Duchenne muscular dystrophy, cognitive disorders, pathogenesis, mutations in dystrophin gene, brain-derived neurotrophic factor (BDNF), nerve growth factor (NGF), ciliary neurotrophic factor (CNTF), immunoenzyme method, blood serum

1. Introduction

Nowadays, researchers have greatly succeeded in understanding the pathogenesis of Duchenne muscular dystrophy (DMD); numerous studies resulted in drugs that can treat some forms of DMD, affecting the course of the disease, converting it from a malignant form to a benign one, and thus increasing locomotion ability of patients

[1]. However, the study of cognitive impairment pathogenesis in DMD patients and a search for drug therapy for these disorders remain an important issue. It is a well-known fact that genetically DMD is caused by mutations in the gene encoding the dystrophin protein, which is a part of the dystrophin-glycoprotein complex and appears both in muscle and nerve cells, being involved in functioning of voltage-dependent channels and in synaptogenesis [2]. The gene encoding the dystrophin protein is the largest human gene, has 5 promoters, has 80 exons, is 24,000 kilobase long, and encodes a 427 kilodaltons protein. [3]. One of the key characteristics of dystrophin is its large number of tissue-specific isoform pairs. So far, researchers have identified more than a dozen isoforms expressed by internal promoters, Dp427, Dp260, Dp140, Dp116, and Dp71, and located in various organs: the lymphocytes, kidneys, cerebral cortex, cerebellum, peripheral nerves, Schwann's sheath, and retina [4–7]. The dystrophin gene has a high frequency of mutations: both point mutations as nucleotide substitutions and extended mutations as deletions and recombinations [8, 9]. Deletions are unevenly distributed along the gene length; they are more likely to be found in hotspots: 50–52 or 42–44 exons. Mutant protein forms in the body lead to dysfunctions of the dystrophin-glycoprotein complex and muscle-nervous system [10]. It is believed that a changed expression of the Dp140 isoform is one of the factors leading to cognitive impairment development in patients with DMD [11]. For example, researchers found that DMD patients with a mutation in promoters of the Dp140 and Dp71 isoforms have IQ index lower than in the case of Dp260 and Dp116 promoter mutations [12]. Still, some researchers associate frequency and severity of mental retardation in DMD patients with the absence of several dystrophin isoforms encoded in the distal end of the gene [13]. Although dystrophin gene mutations have long been recognized as a cause of mental retardation in DMD patients, there are cases when such patients do not have a pronounced cognitive deficit [14].

So, there is still much to be discovered about the occurrence mechanism of cognitive disorders in DMD patients, and some issues are still open to debates. We think that cognitive impairment in DMD patients relies on a combination of mechanisms, leading to a cognitive defect. Among such mechanisms are well-studied molecular genetic factors, distal location of the mutation in the DMD gene or effect from various combinations of impaired synthesis of DMD protein isoforms (Dp140, Dp116, Dp260, and Dp71); on the other hand, none the less important are biochemical factor-associated neurotrophic regulation and apoptosis mechanisms, but these factors are not so well-studied. Regrettably, things we know about physiology of higher nervous activity in terms of neurotrophic regulation are not enough for a comprehensive picture to explain the role of growth neurotrophic factors in cognitive disorder development. However, we know that neurotrophic factors, being polypeptide compounds, are synthesized by neurons and glia cells, get involved in the regulation of growth and differentiation processes, and ensure viability of the nervous tissue and its functions, both in terms of individual neurons and the whole nervous system [15]. Neurotrophins are also involved in synaptic plasticity regulation; they are known to form neuron cytoskeleton, new synapses, and receptors, and they are important for structural ordering of neurons or neuronal groups [16]. Researchers found that polypeptide growth factors are involved in the growth of axons and dendrites, trophic membrane receptors, release of neurotransmitters, and functioning of synapses. So far, the most well-studied neurotrophins, with a very similar structure, are nerve growth factor (NGF) and brain-derived neurotrophic factor (BDNF). Neurotrophic factors also include two subfamilies: glial cell-derived neurotrophic factor (GDNF) and ciliary neurotrophic factor (CNTF). In the human body, neurotrophins are synthesized by a target cell, then diffuse toward the neuron, and bind to receptor molecules on its surface, which causes an active axon growth (sprouting) and dendritic branching (arborization) [17, 18].

So, the axon reaches a target cell and comes into a synaptic contact. Neurotrophins can act both locally, within the same cell population, and remotely, circulating with the blood flow [19]. Neurotrophins make their effect on a neuron through a contact of polypeptide ligands with tyrosine kinase receptors (Trk-A, Trk-B, Trk-C) and low-affinity p75 receptor [20–22]. Neurotrophins trigger a regulating mechanism of cell growth and differentiation by activating a protein kinase cascade called mitogen-activated protein kinase, the MAP kinase pathway [23]. The pathway is activated by Grb2 tyrosine phosphorylation; the Grb2 is a protein that contains SH2 and S3 domains (sre homology region). After a series of cascading reactions, the phosphorylated MAP kinase goes through a nuclear membrane and phosphorylates various gene transcription factors in the nucleus. The resulting gene transcription changes trigger proliferation, differentiation, and maintenance of neuron viability.

NGF is a trophic factor essential for survival and differentiation of nerve cells in the central and peripheral nervous system; it binds to the low-affinity p140 receptor and the high-affinity tyrosine kinase receptor (Trk-A). Myocytes and neurons serve as target cells and secrete neurotrophin, which then binds to receptor ligands on the cell surface, gets captured by a neuron, undergoes endocytosis, and gets retrogradely transported to the nerve cell soma. There, NGF directly affects the nucleus, by changing the generation of enzymes in charge of neurotransmitter synthesis and axon growth.

BDNF is a dimer with a total molecular weight of 27.2 kDa; its structure is similar to that of NGF. Like other neurotrophins, BDNF is involved in the development and survival of brain neurons, including sensory neurons, dopaminergic neurons of the substantia nigra, and cholinergic neurons of the forebrain, hippocampus, and retinal ganglia. Researchers found both mature BDNF forms and pro-BDNF precursors in the central nervous system [24]. It is interesting to study the relations of BDNF expression to the activity of glutamate receptors, commonly found in the central nervous system. It is supposed that BDNF controls the balance between glutamate and (GABA)-ergic systems and has multiple other functions; for instance, when the nervous system is developed, BDNF is involved in synapse formation as well as differentiation, maturation, and survival of neurons.

CNTF is a single-chain polypeptide with 200 amino acid residues and has a molecular weight of 22.7 kDa. It is involved in the survival and differentiation of nervous system cells. High concentrations of CNTF can cause apoptosis. Some researchers believe that CNTF is also involved in glial cell differentiation.

There are many researches that prove that growth polypeptides can be treated as key regulators of cognitive functions and memory retaining processes. Recently, it has been positively proven that NTF growth factors introduced into the brain parenchyma ensure the preservation of brain tissue in critical periods, by protecting neurons from the damaging effects of destructive agents [25–28].

2. Materials and methods

Our research clarified the role of growth factors and apoptosis proteins in cognitive disorder pathogenesis in patients with Duchenne muscular dystrophy. There were 36 male DMD patients aged 5–22 years (average age was 13.7 years) followed up by us in the clinic of North-Western State Medical University named after I.I. Mechnikov, in a stationary unit, and as part of the on-call service of the Saint Petersburg Children's Hospice. The control group consisted of 30 healthy people (7–22 years old, average age 13.8 years). Clinical, molecular genetic, and laboratory tests were carried out. The clinical and neurological examination was conducted according to a generally accepted protocol with inclusion of neuropsychological testing to determine the severity of cognitive disorders. The following methods were used to test the memory: the method of memorizing 10 words; memorizing 9 geometric shapes; delayed reproduction of 10 words and 9 geometric shapes; and Muchnik-Smirnov "double test." Two methods were used for the thinking test, "comparison of concepts" and "directed verbal associations"; attention tests were performed using Schulte tables. We used adapted methods taking into account the age characteristics of DMD patients using a scoring system: memory, attention, and thinking were evaluated from 1 to 30 points, and then the test results were summed up. It helped to differentiate the identified cognitive disorders based on their severity into moderate and severe cognitive disorders (from 1 to 30 points, severe cognitive disorders; from 31 to 60, moderate disorders; and from 61 points to 90 points, no disorders). The search for deletions in the dystrophin gene was performed using multiplex PCR (20 exons and a promoter region). The search for deletions and duplications was performed using multiplex ligation-dependent probe amplification (79 exons and a promoter region). We used sets of probes P034 and P035 by MRC Holland (the Netherlands). The analysis was performed using an automatic capillary electrophoresis system ABI 3130×1 (Applied Biosystems, USA). The detection of point mutations was carried in Cochin Hospital (Paris, France) by next-generation sequencing with subsequent Sanger verification. Determination of the level of neurotrophins and apoptosis proteins is as follows: brain-derived neurotrophic factor, nerve growth factor and ciliary neurotrophic factor (CNTF), caspase 8 (K8), cytochrome C (CC), apoptosis-regulating proteins Bcl2 and p53 were performed using an enzyme immunoassay in blood serum samples. Enzyme immunoassay kits by RayBiotech, Inc. were used. The threshold values for the determination of BGF, NGF, and CNTF were 20 pg/ml, 14 pg/ml, and 8 pg/ml, respectively; K8, 0.10 ng/ml; CC, 0.05 ng/ml; and for Bcl2 and p53 proteins, 0.5 ng/ml and 0.33 U/ml, respectively. DMD patients were divided into two groups based on the presence of cognitive disorders: group 1, patients without cognitive disorders (n = 17); group 2, patients with moderate and severe cognitive disorders (n = 19). In order to clarify the role of the mutation location in the DMD gene, patients with confirmed mutation were divided into two groups based on the location of the mutation in the proximal section of the DMD X chromosome gene (from exon 1 to 40) (n = 8) or the distal section from exon 41 to 79 (n = 16). This distribution was caused by the data on the role of dystrophin protein isoforms expressed from the distal part of the Dp140 and Dp71 genes in the development of cognitive disorders in DMD patients.

The experimental study was carried out in the laboratory of excitable membranes of the FSBES Pavlov Institute of Physiology of the Russian Academy of Sciences. Methods of neural tissue culture, morphometric, immunochemical, and histological studies were used. In order to study the neurotrophic properties of blood plasma in the patients, 5 ml of venous blood was taken on an empty stomach in the morning. The blood was centrifuged, the separated plasma was transferred to a micro-tube and frozen at a temperature of −80°C. The effect of patients' blood plasma on the growth of spinal ganglia neurites was evaluated using the organotypic tissue culture method. An experimental model was based on 10–12-day-old chicken embryos, from which spinal ganglia were isolated at the level of the lumbosacral spine (L5-S1).

Spinal ganglia (explants) were placed on the bottom of a Petri dish covered with a collagen film. Each Petri dish contained 20–25 explants. In order to attach the explants to the collagen substrate, closed Petri dishes were placed in a thermostat at 36.8°C for 10 minutes, and then a nutrient medium was added. We used nutrient media with a pH of 7.4 of the following composition: 40% Hanks solution; 40% Eagle's medium; 15% veal embryonic serum, for cell cultures, HyClone; 5% chicken embryonic extract; with addition of glucose (0.6%), insulin (0.5 u/ml), gentamicin

(100 u/ml), glutamine (0.35%). Chicken embryonic extract was made of 10–12-day-old chicken embryos. Further cultivation of the spinal ganglia explants was performed at 37°C and 5% CO2 for 3 days in a CO2 incubator (Sanyo, Japan).

In order to study the patient's blood plasma parameters and further pharmacological analysis, 25–30 explants per studied concentration were used, taking into account that the experimental test consisted of 10 stages; the average number of explants per patient was 250–300 pieces. Same number of explants was used in the study of blood plasma of healthy people from the control group. Total number of explants studied during the experimental study was 19,000.

When testing blood plasma in tissue culture, blood plasma was added to experimental dishes at the dilution range from 1:100 to 1:2 (1:2, 1:10, 1:50, 1:70, 1:100). Control explants were cultured in a standard nutrient medium without an addition of blood plasma and in a medium with addition of blood plasma of healthy people in the same dilutions. Growth of neurites in tissue culture was studied in vivo using a light microscope and various stains and fluorescent agents. In order to evaluate the growth activity of neurites in the growth zone of the explant and analyze the data obtained, we used a relative criterion—the area index (AI), which was calculated as a ratio of the area of the entire explant, including the peripheral growth zone, to the initial area of the ganglion (AI = S (CA+GA)/S (CA)) (**Figure 1**).

The square of the ocular grid of the microscope was taken as a conventional unit of area (the side of the square at the magnification of 3.5 × 10 was equal to 150 microns). Control AI value was taken as 100%.

In order to clarify the biochemical mechanisms involved in pathological cascades in orphan inherited neuromuscular diseases, a test system was developed that included a sequential study of the patient's blood plasma in an organotypic tissue culture in a 1:70 dilution, followed by an addition of reagents to the medium: synthetic nerve growth factor (100 pg/ml) with subsequent cultivation for 3 days and AI calculation. An indirect immunohistochemical method was used to visualize the cytoskeleton of neurons in the spinal ganglia and their processes (neurites).

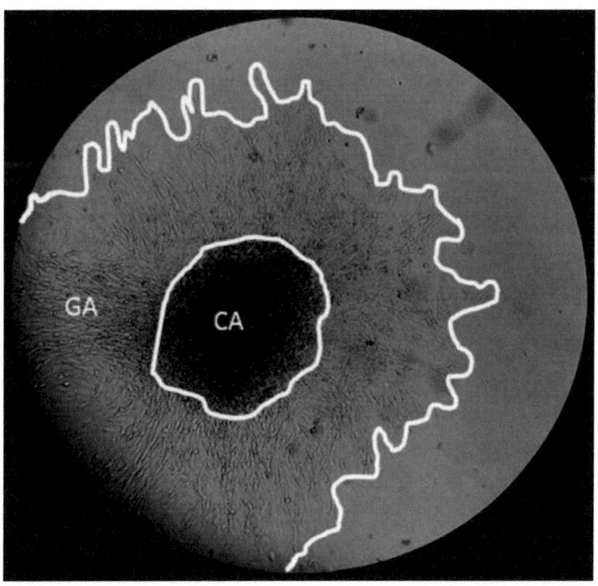

Figure 1.
Diagram of tissue explants of 10–12-day-old chicken embryo (3 days of cultivation) in an organotypic culture. (CA, central area; GA, growth area).

In order to obtain the lifetime information about the condition of cells forming in the growth zone of the spinal ganglia explants and the heart tissues, we used a hardware-software complex for visualization, processing, and analysis of images ZEN_2009 and ZEN_2014 based on laser scanning microscope LSM-710 (Carl Zeiss, Germany). Microscopic tests were performed using an equipment of the Center for Collective Use "confocal microscopy" of the I. P. Pavlov Institute of Physiology of the Russian Academy of Sciences. Visualization of the objects was made using Axiostar Plus microscope (Carl Zeiss, Germany). The resulting images were analyzed using the ImageJ software.

Statistical analysis was performed using STATISTICA 8.0 package (StatSoft®, Inc., USA, 2012). The following methods of statistical analysis were used: assessment of the effect of the quality factor on the variance of the quantitative metric using the analysis of variance, evaluation of the strength and direction of linear association between quantitative variables using parametric Pearson correlation coefficient, nonlinear relationships using Spearman correlation coefficient, conformity assessment according to the Shapiro-Wilk test, and determination of the numerical characteristics of variables. If the null hypothesis was rejected, the median, upper, and lower quartiles of Me [Q25; Q75] were used to test whether the empirical distribution law of a random variable corresponds to the theoretical law of the normal distribution. Quantitative characteristics were described using the arithmetic mean and the standard deviation. The null statistical hypothesis was rejected at a significance level of $p < 0.05$.

3. Results

Thirty-six male patients aged 5–22 years (average age 13.7 years) had Duchenne muscular dystrophy with motor disorders as myopathic syndrome, including generalized muscle weakness, hypotension, as well as pseudohypertrophy. Among the examined DMD patients, 63% had the disease debut at the age of 2–5 years, while 37% had a later onset, at 5–7 years. In 18% of cases, the disease was progressing rapidly, and 13% of patients required mechanical ventilation at the time of study. In all patients, the disease began with damage to muscles of the pelvic girdle and proximal legs and was steadily progressive. All patients had elbow, knee, and ankle joint contractures of varying severity; 56% of patients had spinal deformities of varying severity: scoliosis (25%), kyphoscoliosis (53%), and Friedreich's ataxia deformity. 68% of patients suffered from cardiopathy and 57% of patients from pneumopathy. EDSS scale grades the patients as follows: 22%, high disability degree (9.5 points), bedridden, with a tracheostomy and mechanical ventilation, and requiring full nursing care. 64% ranged from 8.0 to 9.0 EDSS points: they moved in a wheelchair (motorized), retained self-care hand functions, and could independently chew, swallow, and breathe. 10% of patients were graded from 7.0 to 7.5 EDSS points, 4% 6.0–5.5 points. A neuropsychological study found 33% of cases of pronounced cognitive impairment and 19% of moderate cognitive impairment.

A molecular genetic study in DMD patients found genetic polymorphism, with 82% of cases represented by deletion and duplication mutations in the dystrophin protein gene, as 12% by nonsense mutations. Mutations were detected in the DMD gene: most frequent mutations occurred from 43 to 50 exons; (n = 8) patients had mutations in the proximal end of the DMD gene in X chromosome (from 1 to 40 exon); and (n = 18) patients had mutations in the distal end from 41 to 79 exon. Analysis of mutation location in DMD gene showed that synthesis of dystrophin protein isoforms is impaired as follows: Dp260 (n = 18), Dp140 (n = 15), Dp116 (n = 1), and Dp71 (n = 1). 15 patients had the DMD gene mutation in exons that affect synthesis of two isoforms (Dp260 and Dp140) (n = 15) and 1 patient, more than two isoforms (Dp260, Dp140, Dp116, and Dp71) (n = 1). Later, in order to clarify the role of mutation location in the DMD gene, we divided patients with confirmed mutations into two groups—those with mutation located in the proximal end of the DMD gene of X chromosome (from 1 to 40 exon) (n = 8) and those with mutation located the distal end from 41 to 70 exon (n = 16). We noticed that DMD patients with a distal end location of the DMD gene mutation had more pronounced cognitive impairment. However, we received no reliable data about the role of single isoforms of the dystrophin protein in development of cognitive impairment, as there had been insufficient clinical evidence.

In our study of DMD patients, we analyzed blood concentrations of NGF, BDNF, and CNTF growth factors by enzyme immunoassay. BDNF concentration in DMD patients was at a level comparable to the control group, and in some patients BDNF concentration was below the normal level of 21,500 pg/ml [18,650; 23,750] with the normal level of 24,454 [20,380; 29,640]. An enzyme-linked immunosorbent assay showed that serum NGF concentrations in DMD patients are 1,550 pg/ml [864; 1,901] higher than in the control group with 689 pg/ml [365; 987] ($p < 0.001$). CNTF concentration was higher in the blood plasma of DMD patients = 17.8 [12.4; 44.6] than in the control group, with the normal level of 14.9 [11.6; 21.6]. Comparing the concentrations of neurotrophins (NGF, BDNF, CNTF) in DMD patients, divided by the age, we found that patients under 18 showed a statistically significant ($p < 0.001$) excessive concentrations, in comparison with patients over 18. We received statistically significant ($p < 0.05$) results that NGF and BDNF levels are higher in the control group under 18 than in the group over 18. Patients with DMD with a mutation located in the distal end of the dystrophin protein gene (41 to 79 exon) have more pronounced cognitive impairments and a significantly decreased BDNF neurotrophin concentration in blood plasma ($p < 0.01$). DMD patients with cognitive impairment (n = 19) had decreased BDNF concentration of 23,670 [21,700; 30,720] pg/ml vs 32,700 [31,660; 33,750] pg/ml in DMD patients without cognitive impairment. We calculated the absolute risk of DMD with cognitive impairment by BDNF concentration, as well as odds ratios for the risk, and 95% confidence interval for the odds ratios. We divided the BDNF level into two intervals by the pattern of its distribution in the groups under study. **Table 1** shows the absolute risk of DMD with cognitive disorders and odds ratio of this risk, calculated by assessing relations between BDNF concentration and the course of DMD.

Having analyzed the distribution pattern of BDNF concentration in the groups, we identified two groups of patients—≤31,000 pg/ml and >31,000 pg/ml. The minimal risk of DMD with cognitive impairment made 20% (2 out of 10 patients)

BDNF concentration, pg./ml	DMD course without any cognitive disorders		DMD course with development of cognitive disorders		Odds ratio (OR)	95% confidence interval of the odds ratio (CI OR)
	Abs. number	%	Abs. number	%		
>31,000, n = 10	8	80	2	20	*	*
≤31,000, n = 20	5	25	15	75	12.0	1.9–76.4
Total, n = 30	64	42.7	86	57.3		

**The comparison group or the minimum predicted risk group.*

Table 1.
Assessment of the absolute risk of developing cognitive disorders in DMD depending on BDNF concentration.

in the group of patients with BDNF concentration over 31,000 pg/ml. Comparing with the group described above, patients with BDNF concentration less than 31,000 pg/ml had 75% risk of adverse course (15 of 20 patients); and statistically significant ($p < 0.001$) odds for cognitive disorders development were 10 times higher (odds ratio, 12,0; 95% confidence interval for odds ratios, 1.9–76.4).

The study proved that peptide neurotrophic regulation of the central nervous system has a complex nature in a current neurodegenerative process. We found that in DMD concentrations of neurotrophins are comparable to control data and tend to approach the lower normal range. Also, we noted a statistically significant difference in concentrations of neurotrophins (NGF and BDNF) in patients by age: in patients under 18, levels of neurotrophins are higher. This phenomenon can also be explained in terms of theory of neurotrophic neuromuscular interaction during ontogenesis, the key assumption of which is physiological role of neurotrophins synthesized by target cells (neurons and myocytes) to establish synaptic contact with a neuron.

We received controversial results in the laboratory study of patients' blood plasma in terms of content of various peptide substances involved in apoptosis and anti-apoptotic defense mechanisms. Analyzing laboratory results of levels of proteins involved in apoptosis (p53 protein, caspase 8, cytochrome C, Bcl2 protein) in the blood plasma of DMD patients, we found a significant increase in concentration of the proteins in such patients ($p < 0.01$) (**Table 2**).

It should be noted that many peptide substances show pathological activity in the nervous tissue. So, a high content of caspase 8, cytochrome C, p53 protein, and Bcl2 protein in blood of DMD patients indicates massive destruction of muscle tissue. Hyper-production of cytochrome C cannot be treated as a compensatory mechanism, as it is synthesized by mitochondria in the cell and can enter the bloodstream only due to cell destruction, similarly to the creatine phosphokinase enzyme in muscle pathology.

A study of DMD patients' blood plasma in an organotypic culture of nervous tissue showed that blood plasma of the patients has a weak effect on the growth of neurites of spinal ganglia, used as an experimental model. Area index in explants with blood plasma of DMD patients amounts to 105.0 [102.0; 108.0]%, which is less than the area index in the control explants 114.0 [113.0; 115.0] (**Figure 2**). The introduction of synthetic NGF (100 pg/ml) into the organotypic tissue culture with blood plasma of DMD patients increased the area index to 114.0 [111.0; 116.0]%. To explain that situation, we developed the theory of neurotrophic neuromuscular interaction during ontogenesis. In case of DMD, myocytes die, being unable to perform their physiological function not only as a contractile apparatus but also as a target cell. So, in primary muscle damage, synthesis of neurotrophins (NGF, BDNF) decreases.

Regulating proteins	DMD patients	The control group	Criterion Kruskal-Wallis, p
p53, U/ml	17.0 [4.0; 34.0]	0.0 [0.0; 0.4]	<0.001
Bcl2, ng/ml	46.0 [23.0; 87.7]	0.85 [0.0; 2.1]	<0.001
Caspase 8, ng/ml	0.18 [0.14; 0.31]	0.0 [0.0; 0.0]	<0.001
Cytochrome C, ng/ml	0.36 [0.0; 1.6]	0.0 [0.0; 0.0]	<0.001

The results of non-parametric univariate analysis (Kruskal-Wallis ANOVA by ranks).

Table 2.
Concentrations of proteins involved in the process of apoptosis (p53, caspase 8, cytochrome C, and Bcl2 protein) in the blood plasma of patients of the studied groups, $Me[Q_{25}; Q_{75}]$.

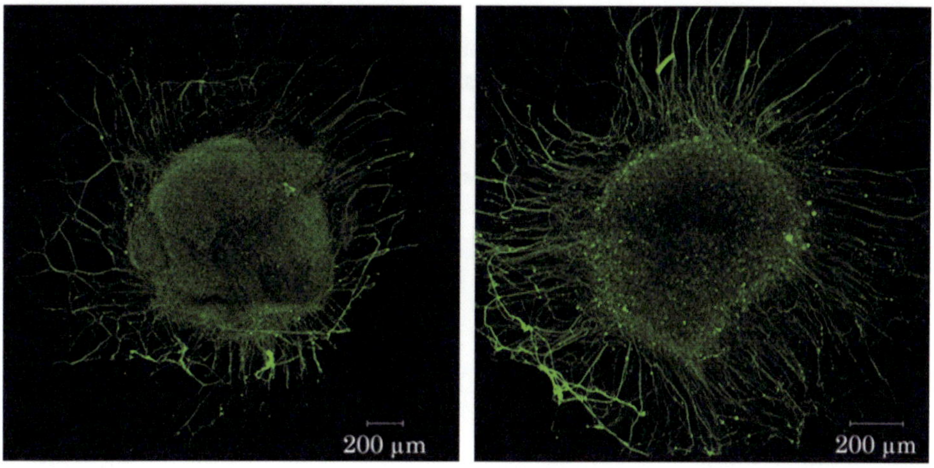

Figure 2.
(a, b) explant of the spinal ganglion of 10–12-day-old chicken embryo (3 days of cultivation) (microphotography). –(a) explant containing blood plasma of DMD patients, dilution (1:70); (b) explant containing blood plasma (control), dilution (1:70).

The clinical and neuropsychological study of DMD patients found cognitive impairments of varying severity in 33% of cases, and most of these patients had mutations of the DMD gene in exons 43–53, i.e., in the distal end. It is worth mentioning that among DMD patients with severe cognitive impairment (n = 4), three patients had a mutation affecting the Dp260 and Dp140 isoforms, and one patient had an impaired synthesis of Dp140, Dp260, Dp116, and Dp71 isoforms. These results prove that there are more pronounced cognitive impairment in DMD patients with a DMD gene mutation that affects synthesis of several DMD protein isoforms; however, we have insufficient clinical data to evaluate the reliability of these results. Analysis of the neurotrophin level in blood plasma in DMD patients shows a complex nature of peptide composition. We found that in the group of DMD patients with cognitive impairment, the concentration of BDNF neurotrophin significantly decreased; and the CNTF level was higher than normal. This may indicate an imbalanced neurotrophic regulation in the central nervous system structures; the imbalance manifests itself in a weakened BDNF effect on the nervous tissue, which results in decreasing rate of differentiation, synaptogenesis, and neuronal growth, on the one hand, and the increasing activity of glial cells, on the other. It causes a decreasing functional activity and dysfunction of neurons and leads to the development of cognitive impairment in DMD patients. However, we still cannot answer the question why it happens in DMD patients with a distal mutation in the dystrophin protein gene. Synthesis of BDNF neurotrophin is encoded on chromosome 11; however, Dp260 and Dp140 isoforms might be necessary for transport or transition from pro-BDNF to the active BDNF form. Perhaps, high concentrations of apoptosis proteins affect the p75 receptor and impair BDNF synthesis. Comparing our results with those of N. Doorenweerd (2014), who studied brain microstructure in DMD patients by quantitative magnetic resonance imaging, we can hypothesize about the role of this factor in cognitive deficiency development in DMD patients [29]. By the Doorenweerd study, DMD patients with an exon mutation of the Dp140(−) isoform and worse results of neuropsychological examination had a smaller brain volume and a smaller amount of gray matter than in the control group and the group of DMD patients with Dp140(+), who showed better results in the examination [30]. A decrease in brain volume may be associated with a low level of BDNF neurotrophin, since we know that this factor stimulates growth and differentiation of brain neurons; however, vice versa supposition may also be valid: a small brain volume synthesizes a smaller amount of BDNF. So, we think that development of cognitive disorders in DMD patients is caused by a number of mechanisms, both of a genetic nature and based on neurotrophic regulation of the nervous system in DMD patients, as well as on secondary factors in terms of increasing activity of apoptosis proteins.

4. Conclusions

Thus, we detected a high content of apoptotic proteins (caspase 8, cytochrome C, p53 protein, and Bcl2 protein) and GNTF neurotrophin, and, at the same time, a reduced concentration of BDNF neurotrophin in blood plasma of DMD patients. In our opinion, this creates an intra-organic chemical imbalance and may serve as one of the factors leading to the development of cognitive impairment in DMD patients, together with such molecular-genetic factors as location of the mutation and impaired synthesis of dystrophin protein isoforms.

Author details

Mariia Georgievna Sokolova[1*] and Ekaterina Valentinovna Lopatina[2]

1 Federal State Budgetary Educational Institution of Higher Education, North-West State Medical University Named After I.I. Mechnikov, of the Ministry of Healthcare of Russian Federation, Saint Petersburg, Russia

2 Federal State Budgetary Educational Institution of Higher Education "Academician I.P. Pavlov First St. Petersburg State Medical University" of the Ministry of Healthcare of Russian Federation, Saint Petersburg, Russia

*Address all correspondence to: sokolova.m08@mail.ru

References

[1] Falzarano MS, Scotton C, Passarelli C. Ferlini a Duchenne muscular dystrophy: From diagnosis to therapy. Molecules. 2015;**20**(10):18168-18184. DOI: 10.3390/molecules201018168

[2] Fuenzalida M, Espinoza C, Pérez MÁ, Tapia-Rojas C, Cuitino L, Brandan E, et al. Wnt signaling pathway improves central inhibitory synaptic transmission in a mouse model of Duchenne muscular dystrophy. Neurobiology of Disease. 2016;**86**:109-120. DOI: 10.1016. /j.nbd.2015.11.018

[3] Leturcq F, Tuffery-Giraud S. Genetics and molecular aspects of dystrophinopathies. Archives de Pédiatrie. 2015;**22**(12 Suppl 1):12S3-12S1211. (Article in French). DOI: 10.1016/S0929-693X(16)30002-1

[4] Miranda R, Nudel U, Laroche S, Vaillend C. Altered presynaptic ultrastructure in excitatory hippocampal synapses of mice lacking dystrophins Dp427 or Dp71. Neurobiology of Disease. 2011;**43**(1):134-141. DOI: 10.1016./j.nbd.2011.02.017

[5] Ricotti V, Jägle H, Theodorou M, Moore AT, Muntoni F, Thompson DA. Ocular and neurodevelopmental features of Duchenne muscular dystrophy: A signature of dystrophin function in the central nervous system. European Journal of Human Genetics. 2016;**24**(4):562-568. DOI: 10.1038/ejhg.2015.135

[6] Fujimoto T, Itoh K, Yaoi T, Fushiki S. Somatodendritic and excitatory postsynaptic distribution of neuron-type dystrophin isoform, Dp40, in hippocampal neurons. Biochemical and Biophysical Research Communications. 2014;**452**(1):79-84. DOI: 10.1016/j.bbrc.2014.08.064

[7] Ramelli GP. Dystrobrevin isoform expression in patients with neuromuscular disease. Clinical Neuropathology. 2010;**29**(4):254-261

[8] Zhong J, Xu T, Chen G, Liao H, Zhang J, Lan D. Genetic analysis of the dystrophin gene in children with Duchenne and Becker muscular dystrophies. Muscle & Nerve. 2017;**56**(1):117-121. DOI: 10.1002/mus

[9] Muntoni F, Torelli S, Ferlini A. Dystrophin and mutations: One gene, several proteins, multiple phenotypes. Lancet Neurology. 2003;**2**(12):731-740

[10] Kim MJ, Cho SI, Chae JH, Lim BC, Lee JS, Lee SJ, et al. Pitfalls of multiple ligation-dependent probe amplifications in detecting DMD exon deletions or duplications. The Journal of Molecular Diagnostics. 2016;**18**(2):253-259. DOI: 10.1016/j.jmoldx.2015.11.002

[11] Taylor PJ, Betts GA, Maroulis S, Gilissen C, Pedersen RL, Mowat DR, et al. Dystrophin gene mutation location and the risk of cognitive impairment in Duchenne muscular dystrophy. PLoS One. 2010;**5**(1):e8803. DOI: 10.1371/journal.pone.0008803

[12] Milic Rasic V, Vojinovic D, Pesovic J, Mijalkovic G, Lukic V, Mladenovic J, et al. Intellectual ability in the duchenne muscular dystrophy and dystrophin gene mutation location. Balkan Journal of Medical Genetics: BJMG. 2015;**17**(2):25-35. DOI: 10.2478/bjmg-2014-0071

[13] Suzuki H, Aoki Y, Kameyama T, Saito T, Masuda S, Tanihata J, et al. Endogenous multiple exon skipping and back-splicing at the DMD mutation hotspot. International Journal of Molecular Sciences. 2016;**17**(10):pii: E1722. DOI: 10.3390/ijms17101722

[14] Anand A, Tyagi R, Mohanty M, Goyal M, Silva KR, Wijekoon N.

Dystrophin induced cognitive impairment: Mechanisms, models and therapeutic strategies. Annals of Neurosciences. 2015;**22**(2):108-118. DOI: 10.5214/ans.0972.7531.221210

[15] Davies AM. The role of neurotrophins in the developing nervous system. Journal of Neurobiology. 1994;**25**(11):1134-1148

[16] Hawryluk GW et al. In vitro characterization of trophic factor expression in neural precursor cells. Stem Cells and Development. 2012;**21**(3):32-47

[17] Matusica D et al. Local versus long-range neurotrophin receptor signalling: Endosomes are not just carriers for axonal transport. Developmental Biology. 2014;**5**:84-95

[18] Siegel S et al. Ciliary neurotrophic factor is required for motoneuron sprouting. Experimental Neurology. 2000;**166**:205-212

[19] Blais M et al. Nerve growth factor, brain-derived neurotrophic factor, neurotrophin-3 and glial-derived neurotrophic factor enhance angiogenesis in a tissue-engineered in vitro model. Tissue Engineering Part A. 2013;**9**:55-64

[20] Chapleau CA et al. Divergent roles of p75NTR and Trk receptors in BDNF's effects on dendritic spine density and morphology. Neural Plasticity. 2012;**3**:27-31

[21] Urbaniak A et al. P75NTR receptor-role in cell growth and apoptosis. Neuroscience. 2013;**19**:312-317

[22] Ventura E et al. Selective targeted delivery of the TNF-alpha receptor p75 and uteroglobin to the vasculature of inflamed tissues: A preliminary report. BMC Biotechnology. 2011;**10**:104-110

[23] Gurgis FM et al. Mitogen-activated protein kinase-activated protein kinase 2 in neuroinflammation, heat shock protein 27 phosphorylation, and cell cycle: Role and targeting. Journal of Neurobiology. 2013;**85**(2):145-156

[24] Brunelli A et al. Acute exercise modulates BDNF and pro-BDNF protein content in immune cells. Medicine and Science in Sports and Exercise. 2012;**44**(10):1771-1777

[25] Wang N et al. Puerarin protected the brain from cerebral ischemia injury via astrocyte apoptosis inhibition. Neuropharmacology. 2014;**70**(4):54-67

[26] Dabidi RV et al. Endurance exercise training and diferuloyl methane supplement: Changes in neurotrophic factor and oxidative stress induced by lead in rat brain. Biology of Sport. 2013;**30**(1):6-10

[27] Slotkin TA et al. Targeting of neurotrophic factors, their receptors, and signaling pathways in the developmental neurotoxicity of organophosphates in vivo and in vitro. Brain Research Bulletin. 2008;**76**(4):24-38

[28] Tonchev AB et al. Brain ischemia, neurogenesis, and neurotrophic receptor expression in primates. Archives Italiennes de Biologie. 2011;**149**(2):25-31

[29] Doorenweerd N, Straathof CS, Dumas EM, Spitali P, Ginjaar IB, Wokke BH, et al. Reduced cerebral gray matter and altered white matter in boys with Duchenne muscular dystrophy. Annals of Neurology. 2014;**76**(3): 403-411. DOI: 10.1002/ana.24222

[30] Doorenweerd N, Dumas EM, Ghariq E, Schmid S, Straathof CS, Roest AA, et al. Kan HE decreased cerebral perfusion in Duchenne muscular dystrophy patients. Neuromuscular Disorders. 2017;**27**(1):29-37. DOI: 10.1016/j.nmd.2016.10.005

Chapter 5

Mesenchymal Stem Cells for Regenerative Medicine for Duchenne Muscular Dystrophy

Ahmed Elhussieny, Ken'ichiro Nogami, Fusako Sakai-Takemura, Yusuke Maruyama, AbdElraouf Omar Abdelbakey, Wael Abou El-kheir, Shin'ichi Takeda and Yuko Miyagoe-Suzuki

Abstract

Mesenchymal stem cells (MSCs) are multipotent stem cells that can be isolated from both foetal and adult tissues. Several groups demonstrated that transplantation of MSCs promoted the regeneration of skeletal muscle and ameliorated muscular dystrophy in animal models. Mesenchymal stem cells in skeletal muscle, also known as fibro-adipogenic progenitors (FAPs), are essential for the maintenance of skeletal muscle. Importantly, they contribute to fibrosis and fat accumulation in dystrophic muscle. Therefore, MSCs in muscle are a pharmacological target for the treatment of muscular dystrophies. In this chapter, we briefly update the knowledge on mesenchymal stem/progenitor cells and discuss their therapeutic potential as a regenerative medicine treatment of Duchenne muscular dystrophy.

Keywords: mesenchymal stem cells, induced pluripotent stem cells, induced MSCs, Duchenne muscular dystrophy, immune response, paracrine factors, cell transplantation, muscle regeneration, dystrophin, satellite cells, inflammation, skeletal muscle, fibrosis, adipocyte

1. Introduction

Duchenne muscular dystrophy (DMD) is an X-linked progressive muscle wasting disorder caused by mutations in the DMD gene [1, 2], affecting 1 in 3500–5000 male births. Serum creatine kinase (CK) levels are elevated at birth, and motor milestones are delayed. Reduced motor skills between age 3 and 5 years provoke diagnostic evaluation. Quality of life for boys with DMD is further affected early in life, with the inability to keep up with peers of early school age and loss of ambulation by 12 years of age; premature death occurs at 20–30 years of age due to respiratory and cardiac complications (https://www.duchenne.com/about-duchenne; https://ghr.nlm.nih.gov/condition/duchenne-and-becker-muscular-dystrophy).

Mutations of the DMD gene cause complete (Duchenne) or partial (Becker) loss of dystrophin protein at the sarcolemma [3]. In normal muscle cells, dystrophin forms a complex with glycoproteins at the sarcolemma, forming a critical link between the extracellular matrix (ECM) and the cytoskeleton [4]. Without the complex, the sarcolemma becomes fragile and is easily disrupted by mechanical stress [4, 5].

Except for corticosteroids, there is currently no effective treatment for DMD [6]. In this chapter, we discuss the potential of mesenchymal stem cells as a therapeutic tool for DMD patients. Many researchers prefer the term 'mesenchymal stromal cells' or 'mesenchymal progenitors' to mesenchymal stem cells because mesenchymal stem cells with self-renewal and trilineage differentiation potential are a minor subpopulation in tissue-derived primary cultures of mesenchymal cells. In this chapter, however, we uniformly refer to them as mesenchymal stem cells.

2. The pathological changes in DMD muscle

The absence of dystrophin causes loss of the dystrophin-associated protein complex (DAPC) at the sarcolemma. The sarcolemma lacking the complex becomes vulnerable to mechanical stress. In addition, signalling through dystrophin-DAPC-associated molecules such as nNOS is disturbed [4, 5]. As a result, myofibres die in large numbers by contraction-induced mechanical stress, and to regenerate injured myofibres, inflammatory cells begin to remove debris of the muscle tissue; at the same time, muscle satellite cells are activated, proliferate and fuse with damaged myofibres. In the case of DMD, however, the cycle of degeneration and regeneration of myofibres repeats throughout life. Therefore, secondary pathological changes gradually develop, including perturbation of calcium homeostasis, activation of Ca^{2+}-dependent proteases, mitochondrial dysfunction in myofibres, impaired regeneration of myofibres due to exhaustion of satellite cells, prolonged inflammation, disturbed immune response, fibrosis and fatty infiltration, with poor vascular adaptation and functional ischaemia [6]. These secondary pathological changes accelerate the disease course of DMD, resulting in severe loss of myofibres and

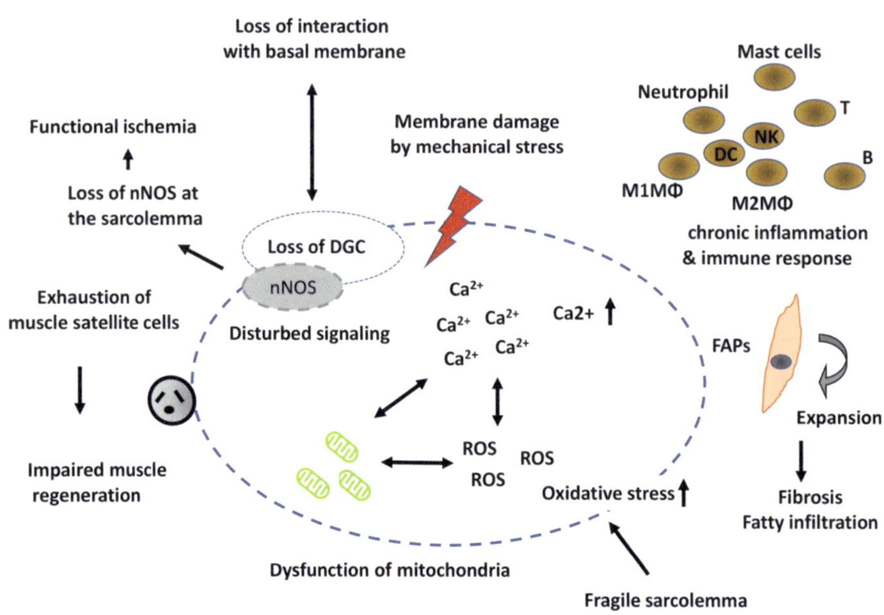

Figure 1.
Deficiency of dystrophin protein at the sarcolemma causes multiple pathological changes in DMD muscle [6, 7].

muscle atrophy. Therefore, in addition to the restoration of dystrophin protein by gene therapy or stem cell therapy, blockage of secondary pathological events is an important therapeutic strategy for DMD (**Figure 1**).

3. Muscle stem cells as a cell-based therapy for DMD

Upon injury, muscle satellite cells are activated, proliferate, and either fuse with damaged myofibres or fuse with each other to form new myofibres [8]. In DMD muscle, satellite cells compensate for muscle fibre loss in the early stages of the disease but eventually are exhausted. As a result, in DMD muscle, the myofibres are gradually replaced with fibrous and fatty connective tissue. Therefore, stem cell transplantation is expected to be a potential therapy for DMD [9].

There are different kinds of stem cells with myogenic potential in skeletal muscle. Muscle satellite cells are authentic unipotent skeletal muscle-specific stem cells [8]. Muscle-derived stem cells (MDSCs) [10] and mesangioblasts [11] were reported to be multipotent and transplantable *via* circulation; therefore, they are expected to be promising tools for cell-based therapies for DMD. Recently, muscle progenitors were induced from pluripotent stem cells as a cell source for cell-based therapy of DMD because induced pluripotent stem cells (iPSCs) can be expanded without losing pluripotency [12]. Myogenic cells induced from iPSCs are usually at a foetal stage and poorly engraft in the muscle of immunodeficient DMD model mice [13, 14].

In addition, muscles affected by muscular dystrophies are in a state of continuous inflammation and are characterised by marked and sustained infiltration of inflammatory and immune cells with fibrosis and adipose replacement. Such pathological microenvironments would not support survival, proliferation, and differentiation of the transplanted stem cells. Therefore, researchers have started to consider not only the properties of stem cells but also the microenvironment.

4. Muscle-resident mesenchymal stem cells (progenitors) are indispensable for muscle homeostasis

Skeletal muscle regenerates when it is injured. The regeneration process is complex but well organised, depending on the interaction among different types of cells: muscle stem/progenitor cells, muscle-resident mesenchymal progenitors and cells involved in inflammatory and innate and adaptive immune responses. Dynamic extracellular matrix (ECM) remodelling is also required for successful muscle regeneration. In the case of a minor traumatic injury, muscle regeneration is rapidly completed by the interplay of these cells. In muscular dystrophies, however, the degeneration/regeneration process is repeated for a long time, causing exhaustion of muscle satellite cells and finally resulting in severe atrophy of skeletal muscles with a loss of myofibres and extensive fibrosis and fat deposition [15].

Fibro/adipogenic progenitors (FAPs) are tissue-resident mesenchymal stem (or stromal or progenitor) cells [16, 17]. Recently, the necessity of FAPs for skeletal muscle regeneration and maintenance was demonstrated using mouse models [18]. The authors demonstrated that depletion of FAPs resulted in loss of expansion of muscle stem cells (MuSCs) and haematopoietic cells after injury and impaired skeletal muscle regeneration [18]. Furthermore, FAP-depleted mice under homeostatic conditions exhibited muscle atrophy and a loss of MuSCs, revealing that FAPs are essential for long-term homeostatic maintenance of skeletal muscle and the MuSC pool [18].

FAPs have dual functions [19, 20]. In small-scale traumatic muscle injury, they are activated, expand and promote muscle regeneration. When regeneration is completed, FAPs are cleared from the regenerated muscle. In pathological conditions, such as muscular dystrophies, they continue to proliferate and contribute to fibrosis and fatty tissue accumulation.

How is the fate of FAPs regulated? Apparently, FAPs are regulated by signals from myogenic cells and immune cells. Altered signals from these cells in dystrophic muscle change the pro-regenerative FAPs to fibrotic and adipogenic types. Recently, Hogarth et al. reported that annexin A2 accumulation in the myofibre matrix promotes adipogenic replacement of FAPs in dysferlin-deficient LGMD2B model mice. The authors also showed that an MMP-14 inhibitor, Batimastat, inhibited adipogenesis of FAP. The authors speculate that Annexin A2 and MMP-14 both prolong the inflammatory environment, therefore causing excessive expansion of FAP in diseased muscle [21]. Pharmacological inhibition of FAP expansion may be a good strategy to prevent fibro/adipogenic changes in dystrophic muscles.

The signals that regulate FAPs remain largely unclear. Interestingly, treating FAPs of young *mdx* mice with trichostatin A (TSA), a histone deacetylase inhibitor, blocked their fibrotic and adipogenic differentiation and promoted a myogenic fate [22] by changing chromatin structure [23]. TSA treatment decreased the expression of adipogenic genes and upregulated myogenic genes in FAPs [22].

5. Inflammation and immune responses in muscular dystrophies

Inflammatory and immune cells (neutrophils, eosinophils, basophils, macrophage NK cells, dendritic cells, T cells, B cells, etc.) are key regulators of muscle regeneration. In particular, macrophages orchestrate the regeneration process. In the early phase of muscle regeneration, M1 (inflammatory) macrophages remove necrotic tissues by phagocytosis and inhibit fusion of myogenic precursor cells. In the later stage, M2 (regulatory) macrophages gradually replace M1 macrophages and play anti-inflammatory and pro-regenerating roles by promoting the differentiation of myogenic cells and the neovascularization of regenerating muscle regeneration [24].

DMD muscle, which remains dystrophin-deficient, experiences continuous cycles of necrosis and regeneration of myofibres. This causes chronic inflammation and evokes T cell-mediated immune responses, which involves the coexistence of both M1 and M2 macrophages and T cells in the muscle, and it further damages myofibres and exacerbates fibrosis and adipocyte infiltration [6, 25, 26]. Therefore, pharmacological inhibition of excess inflammation and immune response is a reasonable therapeutic strategy for DMD.

6. Mesenchymal stem cells as a therapeutic tool for DMD

As a therapeutic tool for regenerative medicine, mesenchymal stem cells (MSCs) have received significant attention in the recent years due to their high growth potential, paracrine effects, immunomodulatory function and few reported adverse effects [27, 28]. Since MSCs show relatively low immunogenicity due to low expression of major histocompatibility (MHC) antigens and their immunomodulation function, they are being used even in allogeneic settings.

6.1 Definition

To facilitate research on MSCs, the International Society of Cellular Therapy (ISCT) formulated minimal criteria for defining multipotent MSCs in 2006 [29]. First, MSCs must be plastic adherent when maintained in standard culture conditions. Second, MSCs must express CD105, CD73 and CD90 and must not express CD45, CD34, CD14, CD11b, CD79alpha, CD19 and HLA-DR surface molecules. Third, MSCs must differentiate into osteoblasts, adipocytes and chondrocytes under standard in vitro differentiation protocols [29].

6.2 Preparation

Historically, MSCs were isolated from bone marrow [30–33]. Currently, MSCs are shown to exist in the perivascular niche in nearly all tissues and are prepared from a variety of tissues, such as the umbilical cord [34], placenta [35], adipose tissue [36] and dental tissues [37]. Preparation of MSCs from those tissues is less invasive than it is from BM. MSCs from different tissues have similar functions, but detailed comparative studies revealed that MSCs of different origins possess different properties [38].

6.3 Differentiation

MSCs are multipotent stem cells that undergo self-renewal and differentiate into multiple tissues of the mesenchymal lineage and into a non-mesenchymal lineage, including neurons, glia, endothelial cells, hepatocytes and β cells in the pancreas [27]. This wide range of differentiation capacities is one reason why mesenchymal stem cells are being tested in almost 1000 clinical trials in regenerative medicine for the musculoskeletal system, nervous system, myocardium, liver, skin and immune diseases (http://ClinicalTrial.gov). Importantly, the differentiation potential of MSCs varies according to their origin, method of isolation and in vitro propagation procedures [39–41].

6.4 Secretome of MSCs

MSCs secrete a variety of bioactive molecules, such as growth factors, chemokines and cytokines. These molecules regulate the survival, proliferation and differentiation of target cells, promote angiogenesis and tissue repair and modulate inflammation and innate or acquired immunity. It is widely accepted that the therapeutic effects of MSCs in preclinical and clinical trials are largely due to their paracrine function [27]. Importantly, the secretome of MSCs varies depending on the age of the donor and the niches where the cells reside [42]. Therefore, it is expected that the therapeutic effects of MSCs with different origins exert will be different.

6.5 Transplanted MSCs ameliorate dystrophic phenotypes of DMD muscle?

6.5.1 Mechanisms of amelioration of the dystrophic phenotype by MSCs

Recently, there has been considerable interest in the clinical application of MSCs for the treatment of muscle diseases. However, the myogenic potential of MSCs is controversial.

Sassoli et al. found that myoblast proliferation was greatly enhanced in coculture with bone marrow MSCs [43]. Myoblasts after coculture expressed higher levels of

Notch-1, a key determinant of myoblast activation and proliferation. Interestingly, the effects were mediated by vascular endothelial growth factor (VEGF) secreted by MSCs [43]. A VEGFR2 inhibitor, KRN633, inhibited the positive effects of MSC-CM on C2C12 cell growth and Notch-1 signalling [43]. Linard et al. showed successful regeneration of rump muscle by local transplantation of bone marrow MSCs (BM-MSCs) after severe radiation burn using a pig model [44]. The authors speculate that locally injected BM-MSCs secreted growth factors such as VEGF and promoted angiogenesis. The authors also showed that MSCs supported the maintenance of the satellite cell pool and created a good macrophage M1/M2 balance. Nakamura et al. reported that transplantation of MSCs promoted the regeneration of skeletal muscle in a rat injury model without differentiation into skeletal myofibres. The report suggests that MSCs contribute to the regeneration of skeletal muscle by paracrine mechanisms [45]. Maeda et al. reported that BM-MSCs transplanted into peritoneal cavities of dystrophin/utrophin double-knockout (dko) mice strongly suppressed dystrophic pathology and extended the lifespan of treated mice [46]. The authors speculated that CXCL12 and osteopontin from BM-MSCs improved muscle regeneration. Bouglé et al. also reported that human adipose-derived MSCs improved the muscle phenotype of DMD mice *via* the paracrine effects of MSCs [47].

In addition to soluble factors, recent studies demonstrated that MSCs secrete a large number of exosomes for intercellular communication [48, 49]. These exosomes are now expected to be a therapeutic tool for many diseases [50, 51]. Nakamura et al. reported that exosomes from MSCs contained miRNAs that promoted muscle regeneration and reduced the fibrotic area [45]. Bier et al. reported that intramuscular transplantation of PL-MSCs in *mdx* mice decreased the serum CK level, reduced fibrosis in the diaphragm and cardiac muscles and inhibited inflammation, partly *via* exosomal miR-29c [49]. Thus, MSC exosomes or MSC cytokines may provide a cell-free therapeutic strategy as an alternative to transplanting MSCs.

On the other hand, Saito et al. reported that BM-MSCs and periosteum MSCs differentiated into myofibres and restored dystrophin expression in *mdx* mice, although the efficiency was low (3%) [52]. Liu et al. showed that FLK-1^{+} adipose-derived MSCs restored dystrophin expression in *mdx* mice [53]. Feng et al. reported that intravenously delivered BM-MSCs increased dystrophin expression in *mdx* mice [54]. Vieira et al. reported that intravenously injected human adipose-derived MSCs successfully reached the muscle of golden retriever muscular dystrophy (GRMD) dogs and that they expressed human dystrophin [55]. Furthermore, Park et al. reported that human tonsil-derived MSCs (T-MSCs) differentiated into myogenic cells in vitro, and transplantation promoted the recovery of muscle function, as demonstrated by gait assessment (footprint analysis); furthermore, such treatment restored the shape of skeletal muscle in mice with a partial myectomy of the gastrocnemius muscle [56]. These reports suggest that MSCs directly contribute to the regeneration of myofibres and restore dystrophin expression.

7. MSCs regulate inflammation and the immune response in muscular dystrophies

In response to damage signals, perivascular MSCs are activated and recruit inflammatory and immune cells and promote inflammation. At a later stage, MSCs begin to suppress inflammation and the immune response. On the other hand, MSCs in circulation are reported to selectively home towards damaged tissue [57]. Once homed, the inflammatory environment stimulates MSCs to produce a large amount of bioactive molecules or to directly interact with inflammatory and immune cells to regulate inflammation and the immune response.

The therapeutic effects of MSCs in preclinical or clinical trials are thought to be partly the result of modulation of innate and adaptive immunity [27], especially through monocyte/macrophage modulation [28]. Inflammation and immune response are part of the pathology of DMD muscle. Therefore, the immunomodulatory functions of MSCs might be useful for the treatment of DMD.

MSCs are supposed to modulate inflammation and the immune response by (a) suppressing the maturation and function of dendritic cells [58–60], (b) promoting macrophage differentiation towards an M2-like phenotype with high tissue remodelling potential and anti-inflammatory activity [61], (c) inhibiting Th17 generation and function [62, 63], (d) inhibiting Th1 cell generation [64], (e) suppressing NK [65, 66] and T cytotoxic cell function [66], (f) stimulating the generation of Th2 cells [67] and (g) inducing Treg cells [64, 66, 68].

Pinheiro et al. investigated the effects of adipose-derived mesenchymal stem cell (AD-MSC) transplantation on dystrophin-deficient mice. Local injection of AD-MSCs improved histological phenotypes and muscle function [69]. AD-MSCs decreased the muscle content of TNF-α, IL-6, TGF-β1 and oxidative stress but increased the levels of VEGF, IL-10 and IL-4 [69]. MSC-derived IL-4 and IL-10 are reported to convert M1 (pro-inflammatory) macrophages to the M2 (anti-inflammatory) type and promote satellite cell differentiation [70]. These results suggest that transplanted AD-MSCs ameliorated the dystrophic phenotype partly by modulating inflammation.

7.1 Suppression of the immune response by MSCs potentiates gene therapy and cell-based therapy

In a clinical trial of gene therapy using a dystrophin transgene, T cells specific to epitopes of pre-existing dystrophin in revertant fibres were detected, suggesting the existence of autoreactive T-cell immunity against dystrophin before treatment [71]. Currently, exon skipping therapy to restore the reading frame of the DMD gene, and readthrough therapy of premature stop codons (e.g. aminoglycosides or ataluren), is being tested in patients with DMD. The treated patients start to produce dystrophin, which provides new epitopes to them. Suppression of undesirable immune responses against newly produced dystrophin might improve the efficiency of gene therapy.

Transplantation of myogenic cells also evokes innate and acquired immune responses against transplanted cells in the recipient. Therefore, immunosuppression by MSCs is expected to improve the engraftment of transplanted cells and the therapeutic effects of cell therapy. In addition, MSCs support the survival, proliferation, migration and differentiation of myogenic cells by secreting trophic factors.

8. Mesenchymal stem cells induced from pluripotent stem cells (iPSCs)

8.1 MSC-like cells induced from human pluripotent stem cells (iMSCs) have properties that are different from tissue MSCs

Although BM-MSCs are well studied and widely tested in regenerative medicine, the collection procedure for bone marrow is invasive and painful. In addition, adult BM-MSCs cannot be expanded in culture beyond 10 passages [72]. To obtain MSCs with higher proliferative potential, other sources of MSCs are gaining attention, such as the umbilical cord and the placenta. MSCs from these sources proliferate better than BM-MSCs but still show limited proliferative activity [38].

hiPSCs can be expanded in vitro without loss of pluripotency and are therefore an ideal source for deriving mesenchymal stem cells of high quality in a large quantity [73–75]. In addition, unlike human ES cells, iPSCs are not accompanied by ethical concerns. To date, many protocols have been reported for the deviation of mesenchymal stem cells from human ES cells/iPS cells [73–77], although the difference in properties among iMSCs induced by different protocols remains to be determined [73, 74, 77]. For clinical use, iMSCs would be generated from well-characterised, pathogen-free, banked iPSCs with known HLA types or from patient-specific iPSCs.

8.2 Are MSCs induced from human pluripotent stem cells (iMSCs) ideal for clinical use?

MSCs induced from human iPS cells are generally characterised as reprogrammed, rejuvenated MSCs with high proliferative activity [78]. A previous study reported that MSCs from human iPSCs could be expanded for approximately 40 passages (120 population doublings) without obvious loss of plasticity or onset of replicative senescence [79]. In addition, iMSCs have been shown to exhibit potent immune-modulatory function and therapeutic properties (**Table 1**) [83]. Spitzhorn et al. reported that iMSCs did not form tumours after transplantation into the liver [84], but to exclude residual undifferentiated iPS cells, purification of MSCs by FACS using MSC markers and careful evaluation of the risk of tumour formation would be required for each preparation.

	BM-MSCs	**Induced MSCs from ES/iPS cells**
Preparation	Autologous or allogeneic, invasive	Many protocols for deviation scale-up production [73–77]
Proliferation	Limited expansion	Proliferate faster, greater proliferation capacity
Senescence	Faster	Slower
Quality	Inconsistent, heterogeneous depend on donor age [80] and health condition, and culture condition	Controllable? Closer to foetal MSCs less mature than tissue-derived MSCs
Differentiation	Trilineage (adipocytes, osteocytes and chondrocytes); hardly differentiate into skeletal muscle	Higher osteogenic differentiation [74]; poor differentiation into adipogenic cells [81]
Stemness	Lost with expansion	Kept for long culture
Safety	No tumour formation; pathogens from the donors	Genomic instability during the expansion of iPSCs; tumorigenic potential by residual hiPSCs
Paracrine effects	Inhibit apoptosis, promote proliferation and differentiation of the cells, promote tissue regeneration; different secretome [82]	
Immunomodulation function	Regulate inflammation, innate and acquired immunity	Stronger than BM-MSCs? [74, 83]
Suitable for cell therapy?	Being tested in preclinical and clinical trials without serious side effects	Unlimited source of MSCs; autologous MSCs are available
Genome editing	Difficult	Possible

Table 1.
Comparison of properties of human iMSCs with human BM-MSCs.

8.3 iMSCs for muscle disease

The therapeutic potential of iMSCs has been tested in bone regeneration [83, 85], intestinal healing [86], myocardial disorders [82, 87], limb ischaemia [79] and autoimmune disease [88, 89]. In these studies, iMSCs showed therapeutic effects that were comparable or superior to those of tissue MSCs. In the muscular dystrophy field, there are only a small number of reports so far. Jeong et al. reported that iMSCs transplanted into the tibialis anterior of *mdx* mice decreased oxidative damage, as evidenced by a reduction in nitrotyrosine levels, and achieved normal dystrophin expression levels [90]. Since direct differentiation of MSCs into myogenic cells is generally limited, the observed effects of iMSCs might be due to the secretion of bioactive molecules that exert immunomodulatory effects and provide trophic support to myogenic cells.

Importantly, however, Liu et al. recently reported that transplantation of BM-MSCs from C57BL/6 mice aggravated inflammation, oxidative stress and fibrosis and impaired regeneration of contusion-injured C57/Bl6 muscle [91]. Although the mechanisms are not clear, the microenvironment in contusion-damaged muscle might induce the transformation of MSCs into the fibrotic phenotype. Caution might be warranted in the clinical application of MSCs to highly fibrotic muscle.

9. Conclusions

MSCs are multifunctional cells. MSCs secrete trophic factors that help regenerate myofibres. In addition, MSCs suppress inflammation and the immune response in dystrophic mice to protect muscle. MSCs are also expected to support the engraftment of transplanted myogenic cells in recipient muscle. Fortunately, recent technology gives us an option to derive MSC-like cells from pluripotent stem cells. Thus, MSCs are a promising next-generation tool for cell-based therapy of DMD (**Figure 2**).

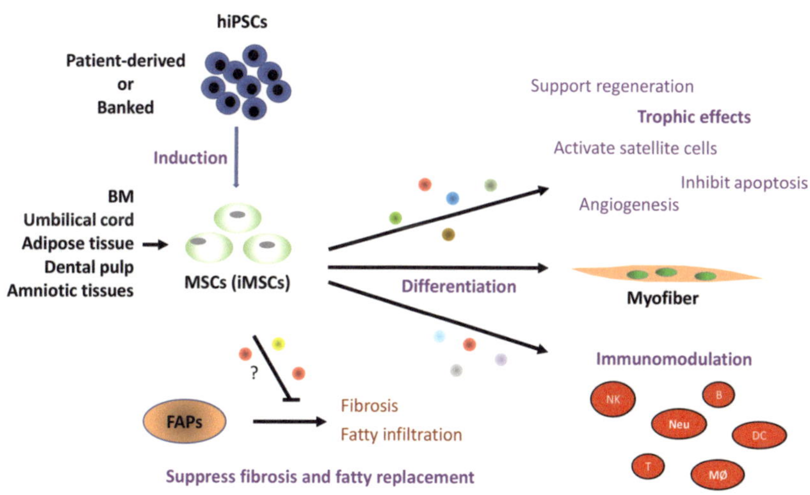

Figure 2.
Mesenchymal stem cells ameliorate the dystrophic phenotype of DMD muscle. Mesenchymal stem-like cells can be derived from human iPSCs (iMSCs). MSCs, which arrive in the muscle either through direction transplantation or via *circulation, secrete a variety of bioactive molecules that promote angiogenesis and support the proliferation and differentiation of satellite cells, thereby promoting muscle regeneration. MSCs also suppress excess inflammatory and immune responses. Whether transplanted MSCs can directly modulate the phenotype of FAPs (resident MSCs) to inhibit fibrosis and fatty replacement remains to be determined. Abbreviations: DC, dendritic cells; NK, natural killer cells; Neu, neutrophil; Mø, macrophage; T, T lymphocytes; B, B lymphocyte.*

Acknowledgements

A.E. is supported by the Channel System Program (CPS) of the Egyptian and Japanese governments. This study was supported by (1) 'Research on refractory musculoskeletal diseases using disease-specific induced pluripotent stem (iPS) cells' from the Research Center Network for Realization of Regenerative Medicine, Japan Agency for Medical Research and Development (AMED), (2) Grants-in-aid for Scientific Research (C) (16K08725 and 19K075190001) from the Ministry of Education, Culture, Sports, Science and Technology (MEXT), Japan and (3) Intramural Research Grants (30-9) for Neurological and Psychiatric Disorders of NCNP.

Conflict of interest

The authors declare no conflicts of interest.

Author details

Ahmed Elhussieny[1,2], Ken'ichiro Nogami[1,3], Fusako Sakai-Takemura[1], Yusuke Maruyama[1,4], AbdElraouf Omar Abdelbakey[2], Wael Abou El-kheir[5], Shin'ichi Takeda[1] and Yuko Miyagoe-Suzuki[1]*

1 Department of Molecular Therapy, National Institute of Neuroscience, National Center of Neurology and Psychiatry, Kodaira, Tokyo, Japan

2 Department of Neurology, Faculty of Medicine, Minia University, Minia, Egypt

3 Department of Neurology, Neurological Institute, Graduate School of Medical Sciences, Kyushu University, Fukuoka, Japan

4 Department of Gene Regulation, Faculty of Pharmaceutical Sciences, Tokyo University of Science, Noda, Chiba, Japan

5 Egyptian Military Medical Academy, Cairo, Egypt

*Address all correspondence to: miyagoe@ncnp.go.jp

References

[1] Koenig M, Hoffman EP, Bertelson CJ, et al. Complete cloning of the Duchenne muscular dystrophy (DMD) cDNA and preliminary genomic organization of the DMD gene in normal and affected individuals. Cell. 1987;**50**:509-517. DOI: 10.1016/0092-8674(87)90504-6

[2] Guiraud S, Aartsma-Rus NM, Vieira KE, et al. The pathogenesis and therapy of muscular dystrophies. Annual Review of Genomics and Human Genetics. 2015;**16**:281-308. DOI: 10.1146/annurev-genom-090314-025003

[3] Arahata K, Ishiura S, Ishiguro T, et al. Immunostaining of skeletal and cardiac muscle surface membrane with antibody against Duchenne muscular dystrophy peptide. Nature. 1988;**333**:861-863. DOI: 10.1038/333861a0

[4] Ozawa E. Our trails and trials in the subsarcolemmal cytoskeleton network and muscular dystrophy researches in the dystrophin era. Proceedings of the Japan Academy Series B, Physical and Biological Sciences. 2010;**86**:798-821. DOI: 10.2183/pjab.86.798

[5] Matsumura K, Campbell KP. Dystrophin-glycoprotein complex: Its role in the molecular pathogenesis of muscular dystrophies. Muscle & Nerve. 1994;**17**:2-15. DOI: 10.1002/mus.880170103

[6] Verhaart IEC, Aartsma-Rus A. Therapeutic developments for Duchenne muscular dystrophy. Nature Reviews. Neurology. 2019;**15**:373-386. DOI: 10.1038/s41582-019-0203-3

[7] Tidball JG, Welc SS, Wehling-Henricks M. Immunobiology of inherited muscular dystrophies. Comprehensive Physiology. 2018;**8**:1313-1356. DOI: 10.1002/cphy.c170052

[8] Fukada S. The roles of muscle stem cells in muscle injury, atrophy and hypertrophy. Journal of Biochemistry. 2018;**163**:353-358. DOI: 10.1093/jb/mvy019

[9] Sun C, Serra C, Lee G, Wagner KR. Stem cell-based therapies for Duchenne muscular dystrophy. Experimental Neurology. 2020;**323**:113086. DOI: 10.1016/j.expneurol.2019.113086

[10] Huard J. Stem cells, blood vessels, and angiogenesis as major determinants for musculoskeletal tissue repair. Journal of Orthopaedic Research. 2019;**37**:1212-1220. DOI: 10.1002/jor.24058

[11] Cossu G, Previtali SC, Napolitano S, et al. Intra-arterial transplantation of HLA-matched donor mesoangioblasts in Duchenne muscular dystrophy. EMBO Molecular Medicine. 2015;7:1513-1528. DOI: 10.15252/emmm.201505636

[12] Miyagoe-Suzuki Y, Takeda S. Skeletal muscle generated from induced pluripotent stem cells - Induction and application. World Journal of Stem Cells. 2017;**9**:89-97. DOI: 10.4252/wjsc.v9.i6.89

[13] Hicks MR, Hiserodt J, Paras K, et al. ERBB3 and NGFR mark a distinct skeletal muscle progenitor cell in human development and hPSCs. Nature Cell Biology. 2018;**20**:46-57. DOI: 10.1038/s41556-017-0010-2

[14] Sakai-Takemura F, Narita A, Masuda S, et al. Premyogenic progenitors derived from human pluripotent stem cells expand in floating culture and differentiate into transplantable myogenic progenitors. Scientific Reports. 2018;**8**:6555. DOI: 10.1038/s41598-018-24959-y

[15] Morgan J, Partridge T. Skeletal muscle in health and disease. Disease Models & Mechanisms.

2020;**13**:dmm042192. DOI: 10.1242/dmm.042192

[16] Uezumi A, Fukada S, Yamamoto N, et al. Mesenchymal progenitors distinct from satellite cells contribute to ectopic fat cell formation in skeletal muscle. Nature Cell Biology. 2010;**12**:143-152. DOI: 10.1038/ncb2014

[17] Joe AW, Yi L, Natarajan A, et al. Muscle injury activates resident fibro/adipogenic progenitors that facilitate myogenesis. Nature Cell Biology. 2010;**12**:153-163. DOI: 10.1038/ncb2015

[18] Wosczyna MN, Konishi CT, Perez Carbajal EE, et al. Mesenchymal stromal cells are required for regeneration and homeostatic maintenance of skeletal muscle. Cell Reports. 2019;**27**:2029-2035. DOI: 10.1016/j.celrep.2019.04.074

[19] Uezumi A, Ito T, Morikawa D, et al. Fibrosis and adipogenesis originate from a common mesenchymal progenitor in skeletal muscle. Journal of Cell Science. 2011;**124**:3654-3664. DOI: 10.1242/jcs.086629

[20] Uezumi A, Ikemoto-Uezumi M, Tsuchida K. Roles of nonmyogenic mesenchymal progenitors in pathogenesis and regeneration of skeletal muscle. Review. Frontiers in Physiology. 2014;**5**:68. DOI: 10.3389/fphys.2014.00068

[21] Hogarth MW, Defour A, Lazarski C, et al. Fibroadipogenic progenitors are responsible for muscle loss in limb girdle muscular dystrophy 2B. Nature Communications. 2019;**10**(1):2430. DOI: 10.1038/s41467-019-10438-z

[22] Mozzetta C, Consalvi S, Saccone V, et al. Fibroadipogenic progenitors mediate the ability of HDAC inhibitors to promote regeneration in dystrophic muscles of young, but not old Mdx mice. EMBO Molecular Medicine. 2013;**5**:626-639. DOI: 10.1002/emmm.201202096

[23] Saccone V, Consalvi S, Giordani L, et al. HDAC-regulated myomiRs control BAF60 variant exchange and direct the functional phenotype of fibro-adipogenic progenitors in dystrophic muscles. Genes & Development. 2014;**28**:841-857. DOI: 10.1101/gad.234468.113

[24] Klimczak A, Kozlowska U, Kurpisz M. Muscle stem/progenitor cells and mesenchymal stem cells of bone marrow origin for skeletal muscle regeneration in muscular dystrophies. Archivum Immunologiae et Therapiae Experimentalis. 2018;**6**:341-354. DOI: 10.1007/s00005-018-0509-7

[25] Evans NP, Misyak SA, Robertson JL, et al. Immune-mediated mechanisms potentially regulate the disease time-course of Duchenne muscular dystrophy and provide targets for therapeutic intervention. PM & R: The Journal of Injury, Function, and Rehabilitation. 2009;**1**:755-768. DOI: 10.1016/j.pmrj.2009.04.010

[26] Rosenberg AS, Puig M, Nagaraju K, et al. Immune-mediated pathology in Duchenne muscular dystrophy (review). Science Translational Medicine. 2015;7:299rv4. DOI: 10.1126/scitranslmed.aaa7322

[27] Andrzejewska A, Lukomska B, Janowski M. Concise review: Mesenchymal stem cells: From roots to boost. Stem Cells. 2019;**37**:855-864. DOI: 10.1002/stem.3016

[28] Jiang W, Xu J. Immune modulation by mesenchymal stem cells. Cell Proliferation. 2020;**53**:e12712. DOI: 10.1111/cpr.12712

[29] Dominici M, Le Blanc K, Mueller I, et al. Minimal criteria for defining multipotent mesenchymal stromal cells. The International Society for Cellular Therapy position statement. Cytotherapy. 2006;**8**:315-317. DOI: 10.1080/14653240600855905

[30] Friedenstein AJ, Petrakova KV, Kurolesova AI, Frolova GP. Heterotopic of bone marrow. Analysis of precursor cells for osteogenic and hematopoietic tissues. Transplantation. 1968;**6**:230-247

[31] Friedenstein AJ, Chailakhjan RK, Lalykina KS. The development of fibroblast colonies in monolayer cultures of Guinea-pig bone marrow and spleen cells. Cell and Tissue Kinetics. 1970;**3**:393-403. DOI: 10.1111/j.1365-2184.1970.tb00347.x

[32] Friedenstein AJ, Chailakhyan RK, Latsinik NV, et al. Stromal cells responsible for transferring the microenvironment of the hemopoietic tissues. Cloning in vitro and retransplantation in vivo. Transplantation. 1974;**17**:331-340. DOI: 10.1097/00007890-197404000-00001

[33] Pittenger MF, Mackay AM, Beck SC, et al. Multilineage potential of adult human mesenchymal stem cells. Science. 1999;**284**:143-147. DOI: 10.1126/science.284.5411.143

[34] Bieback K, Kern S, Klüter H, Eichler H. Critical parameters for the isolation of mesenchymal stem cells from umbilical cord blood. Stem Cells. 2004;**22**:625-634. DOI: 10.1634/stemcells.22-4-625

[35] Igura K, Zhang X, Takahashi K, et al. Isolation and characterization of mesenchymal progenitor cells from chorionic villi of human placenta. Cytotherapy. 2004;**6**:543-553. DOI: 10.1080/14653240410005366-1

[36] Katz AJ, Tholpady A, Tholpady SS, et al. Cell surface and transcriptional characterization of human adipose-derived adherent stromal (hADAS) cells. Stem Cells. 2005;**23**:412-423. DOI: 10.1634/stemcells.2004-0021

[37] Gronthos S, Mankani M, Brahim J, et al. Postnatal human dental pulp stem cells (DPSCs) in vitro and in vivo. Proceedings of the National Academy of Sciences of the United States of America. 2000;**97**:13625-13630. DOI: 10.1073/pnas.240309797

[38] Hass R, Kasper C, Böhm S, Jacobs R. Different populations and sources of human mesenchymal stem cells (MSC): A comparison of adult and neonatal tissue-derived MSC. Cell Communication and Signaling: CCS. 2011;**9**:1. DOI: 10.1186/1478-811X-9-12

[39] Phinney DG, Kopen G, Righter W, Webster S, Tremain N, Prockop DJ. Donor variation in the growth properties and osteogenic potential of human marrow stromal cells. Journal of Cellular Biochemistry. 1999;**75**:424-436

[40] Kern S, Eichler H, Stoeve J, et al. Comparative analysis of mesenchymal stem cells from bone marrow, umbilical cord blood, or adipose tissue. Stem Cells. 2006;**24**:1294-1301. DOI: 10.1634/stemcells.2005-0342

[41] Zhou S, Greenberger JS, Epperly MW, et al. Age-related intrinsic changes in human bone-marrow-derived mesenchymal stem cells and their differentiation to osteoblasts. Aging Cell. 2008;**7**:335-343. DOI: 10.1111/j.1474-9726.2008.00377.x

[42] Kumar LP, Kandoi S, Misra R, Vijayalakshmi S, Rajagopal K, Verma RS. The mesenchymal stem cell secretome: A new paradigm towards cell-free therapeutic mode in regenerative medicine. Cytokine & Growth Factor Reviews. 2019;**46**:1-9. DOI: 10.1016/j.cytogfr.2019.04.002

[43] Sassoli C, Pini A, Chellini F, et al. Bone marrow mesenchymal stromal cells stimulate skeletal myoblast proliferation through the paracrine release of VEGF. PLoS One. 2012;**7**:e37512. DOI: 10.1371/journal.pone.0037512

[44] Linard C, Brachet M, L'homme B, et al. Long-term effectiveness of local BM-MSCs for skeletal muscle regeneration: A proof of concept obtained on a pig model of severe radiation burn. Stem Cell Research & Therapy. 2018;**9**:299. DOI: 10.1186/s13287-018-1051-6

[45] Nakamura Y, Miyaki S, Ishitobi H, et al. Mesenchymal-stem-cell-derived exosomes accelerate skeletal muscle regeneration. FEBS Letters. 2015;**589**:1257-1265. DOI: 10.1016/j.febslet.2015.03.031

[46] Maeda Y, Yonemochi Y, Nakajyo Y, et al. CXCL12 and osteopontin from bone marrow-derived mesenchymal stromal cells improve muscle regeneration. Scientific Reports. 2017;**7**:3305. DOI: 10.1038/s41598-017-02928-1

[47] Bouglé A, Rocheteau P, Briand D, et al. Beneficial role of adipose-derived mesenchymal stem cells from microfragmented fat in a murine model of Duchenne muscular dystrophy. Muscle & Nerve. 2019;**60**:328-335. DOI: 10.1002/mus.26614

[48] Phinney DG, Di Giuseppe M, Njah J, et al. Mesenchymal stem cells use extracellular vesicles to outsource mitophagy and shuttle microRNAs. Nature Communications. 2015;**6**:8472. DOI: 10.1038/ncomms9472

[49] Bier A, Berenstein P, Kronfeld N, et al. Placenta-derived mesenchymal stromal cells and their exosomes exert therapeutic effects in Duchenne muscular dystrophy. Biomaterials. 2018;**174**:67-78. DOI: 10.1016/j.biomaterials.2018.04.055

[50] Phinney DG, Pittenger MF. Concise review: MSC-derived exosomes for cell-free therapy. Stem Cells. 2017;**35**:851-858. DOI: 10.1002/stem.2575

[51] Elahi FM, Farwell DG, Nolta JA, Anderson JD. Preclinical translation of exosomes derived from mesenchymal stem/stromal cells. Stem Cells. 2020;**38**:15-21. DOI: 10.1002/stem.3061

[52] Saito T, Dennis JE, Lennon DP, et al. Myogenic expression of mesenchymal stem cells within myotubes of mdx mice in vitro and in vivo. Tissue Engineering. 1995;**1**:327-343. DOI: 10.1089/ten.1995.1.327

[53] Liu Y, Yan X, Sun Z, et al. Flk-1$^+$ adipose-derived mesenchymal stem cells differentiate into skeletal muscle satellite cells and ameliorate muscular dystrophy in mdx mice. Stem Cells and Development. 2007;**16**:695-706. DOI: 10.1089/scd.2006.0118

[54] Feng S-W, Lu X-L, Liu Z-S, et al. Dynamic distribution of bone marrow-derived mesenchymal stromal cells and change of pathology after infusing into mdx mice. Cytotherapy. 2008;**10**:254-264. DOI: 10.1080/14653240802020381

[55] Vieira NM, Valadares M, Zucconi E, et al. Human adipose-derived mesenchymal stromal cells injected systemically into GRMD dogs without immunosuppression are able to reach the host muscle and express human dystrophin. Cell Transplantation. 2012;**21**:1407-1417. DOI: 10.3727/096368911X

[56] Park S, Choi Y, Jung N, et al. Myogenic differentiation potential of human tonsil-derived mesenchymal stem cells and their potential for use to promote skeletal muscle regeneration. International Journal of Molecular Medicine. 2016;**37**:1209-1220. DOI: 10.3892/ijmm.2016.2536

[57] Rustad KC, Gurtner GC. Mesenchymal stem cells home to sites of injury and inflammation. Advances in Wound Care (New Rochelle). 2012;**1**:147-152. DOI: 10.1089/wound.2011.0314

[58] Jiang XX, Zhang Y, Liu B, et al. Human mesenchymal stem cells

inhibit differentiation and function of monocyte-derived dendritic cells. Blood. 2005;**105**:4120-4126. DOI: 10.1182/blood-2004-02-0586

[59] Chen L, Zhang W, Yue H, et al. Effects of human mesenchymal stem cells on the differentiation of dendritic cells from CD34+ cells. Stem Cells and Development. 2007;**16**:719-731. DOI: 10.1089/scd.2007.0065

[60] Spaggiari GM, Abdelrazik H, Becchetti F, Moretta L. MSCs inhibit monocyte-derived DC maturation and function by selectively interfering with the generation of immature DCs: Central role of MSC-derived prostaglandin E2. Blood. 2009;**113**:6576-6583

[61] Luz-Crawford P, Jorgensen C, Djouad F. Mesenchymal stem cells direct the immunological fate of macrophages. Results and Problems in Cell Differentiation. 2017;**62**:61-72. DOI: 10.1007/978-3-319-54090-0_4

[62] Rafei M, Campeau PM, Aguilar-Mahecha A, et al. Mesenchymal stromal cells ameliorate experimental autoimmune encephalomyelitis by inhibiting CD4 Th17 T cells in a CC chemokine ligand 2-dependent manner. Journal of Immunology. 2009;**182**:5994-6002. DOI: 10.4049/jimmunol.0803962

[63] Duffy MM, Pindjakova J, Hanley SA, et al. Mesenchymal stem cell inhibition of T-helper 17 cell-differentiation is triggered by cell-cell contact and mediated by prostaglandin E2 via the EP4 receptor. European Journal of Immunology. 2011;**41**:2840-2851. DOI: 10.1002/eji.201141499

[64] Batten P, Sarathchandra P, Antoniw JW, et al. Human mesenchymal stem cells induce T cell anergy and downregulate T cell Allo-responses via the TH2 pathway: Relevance to tissue engineering human heart valves. Tissue Engineering. 2006;**12**:2263-2273. DOI: 10.1089/ten.2006.12.2263

[65] Spaggiari GM, Capobianco A, Abdelrazik H, et al. Mesenchymal stem cells inhibit natural killer-cell proliferation, cytotoxicity, and cytokine production: Role of indoleamine 2,3-dioxygenase and prostaglandin E2. Blood. 2008;**111**:1327-1333. DOI: 10.1182/blood-2007-02-074997

[66] Selmani Z, Naji A, Zidi I, et al. Human leukocyte antigen-G5 secretion by human mesenchymal stem cells is required to suppress T lymphocyte and natural killer function and to induce $CD4^+CD25^{high}FOXP3^+$ regulatory T cells. Stem Cells. 2008;**26**:212-222. DOI: 10.1634/stemcells.2007-0554

[67] Bai L, Lennon DP, Eaton V, et al. Human bone marrow-derived mesenchymal stem cells induce Th2-polarized immune response and promote endogenous repair in animal models of multiple sclerosis. Glia. 2009;**57**:1192-1203. DOI: 10.1002/glia.20841

[68] Casiraghi F, Azzollini N, Cassis P, et al. Pretransplant infusion of mesenchymal stem cells prolongs the survival of a semiallogeneic heart transplant through the generation of regulatory T cells. Journal of Immunology. 2008;**181**:3933-3946. DOI: 10.4049/jimmunol.181.6.3933

[69] Pinheiro CH, de Queiroz JC, Guimarães-Ferreira L, et al. Local injections of adipose-derived mesenchymal stem cells modulate inflammation and increase angiogenesis ameliorating the dystrophic phenotype in dystrophin-deficient skeletal muscle. Stem Cell Reviews and Reports. 2012;**8**:363-374. DOI: 10.1007/s12015-011-9304-0

[70] Deng B, Wehling-Henricks M, Villalta SA, et al. IL-10 triggers changes in macrophage phenotype

that promote muscle growth and regeneration. Journal of Immunology. 2012;**189**:3669-3680

[71] Mendell JR, Campbell K, Rodino-Klapac L, et al. Dystrophin immunity in Duchenne's muscular dystrophy. The New England Journal of Medicine. 2010;**363**:1429-1437. DOI: 10.1056/NEJMoa1000228

[72] Izadpanah R, Trygg C, Patel B, et al. Biologic properties of mesenchymal stem cells derived from bone marrow and adipose tissue. Journal of Cellular Biochemistry. 2006;**99**:1285-1297. DOI: 10.1002/jcb.20904

[73] Zhao C, Ikeya M. Generation and applications of induced pluripotent stem cell-derived mesenchymal stem cells. Stem Cells International. 2018;**2018**:9601623. DOI: 10.1155/2018/9601623

[74] Dayem AA, Lee SB, Kim K, et al. Production of mesenchymal stem cells through stem cell reprogramming. International Journal of Molecular Sciences. 2019;**20**:1922. DOI: 10.3390/ijms20081922

[75] Jiang B, Yan L, Wang X, et al. Concise review: Mesenchymal stem cells derived from human pluripotent cells, an unlimited and quality-controllable source for therapeutic applications. Stem Cells. 2019;**37**:572-581. DOI: 10.1002/stem.2964

[76] Hynes K, Menicanin D, Mrozik K, et al. Generation of functional mesenchymal stem cells from different induced pluripotent stem cell lines. Stem Cells and Development. 2014;**23**:1084-1096. DOI: 10.1089/scd.2013.0111

[77] Steens J, Klein D. Current strategies to generate human mesenchymal stem cells in vitro. Stem Cells International. 2018;**2018**:6726185. DOI: 10.1155/2018/6726185

[78] Frobel J, Hemeda H, Lenz M, et al. Epigenetic rejuvenation of mesenchymal stromal cells derived from induced pluripotent stem cells. Stem Cell Reports. 2014;**3**:414-422. DOI: 10.1016/j.stemcr.2014.07.003

[79] Lian Q, Zhang Y, Zhang J, et al. Functional mesenchymal stem cells derived from human induced pluripotent stem cells attenuate limb ischemia in mice. Circulation. 2010;**121**:1113-1123. DOI: 10.1161/CIRCULATIONAHA.109.898312

[80] Stolzing A, Jones E, McGonagle D, Scutt A. Age-related changes in human bone marrow-derived mesenchymal stem cells: Consequences for cell therapies. Mechanisms of Ageing and Development. 2008;**129**:163-173. DOI: 10.1016/j.mad.2007.12.002

[81] Kang R, Zhou Y, Tan S, et al. Mesenchymal stem cells derived from human induced pluripotent stem cells retain adequate osteogenicity and chondrogenicity but less adipogenicity. Stem Cell Research & Therapy. 2015;**6**:144. DOI: 10.1186/s13287-015-0137-7

[82] Liang Y, Li X, Zhang Y, et al. Induced pluripotent stem cells-derived mesenchymal stem cells attenuate cigarette smoke-induced cardiac remodeling and dysfunction. Frontiers in Pharmacology. 2017;**8**:501. DOI: 10.3389/fphar.2017.00501

[83] Kimbrel EA, Kouris NA, Yavanian GJ, et al. Mesenchymal stem cell population derived from human pluripotent stem cells displays potent immunomodulatory and therapeutic properties. Stem Cells and Development. 2014;**23**:1611-1624. DOI: 10.1089/scd.2013.0554

[84] Spitzhorn LS, Kordes C, Megges M, et al. Transplanted human pluripotent stem cell-derived mesenchymal stem

cells support liver regeneration in Gunn rats. Stem Cells and Development. 2018;**27**:1702-1714. DOI: 10.1089/scd.2018.0010

[85] Jungbluth P, Spitzhorn LS, Grassmann J, et al. Human iPSC-derived iMSCs improve bone regeneration in mini-pigs. Bone Research. 2019;7:32. DOI: 10.1038/s41413-019-0069-4

[86] Soontararak S, Chow L, Johnson V, et al. Mesenchymal stem cells (MSC) derived from induced pluripotent stem cells (iPSC) equivalent to adipose-derived MSC in promoting intestinal healing and microbiome normalization in mouse inflammatory bowel disease model. Stem Cells Translational Medicine. 2018;7:456-467. DOI: 10.1002/sctm.17-0305

[87] Zhang Y, Liang X, Liao S, et al. Potent paracrine effects of human induced pluripotent stem cell-derived mesenchymal stem cells attenuate doxorubicin-induced cardiomyopathy. Scientific Reports. 2015;**5**:11235. DOI: 10.1038/srep11235

[88] Hao Q, Zhu YG, Monsel A, et al. Study of bone marrow and embryonic stem cell-derived human mesenchymal stem cells for treatment of *Escherichia coli* endotoxin-induced acute lung injury in mice. Stem Cells Translational Medicine. 2015;**4**:832-840. DOI: 10.5966/sctm.2015-0006

[89] Ferrer L, Kimbrel EA, Lam A, et al. Treatment of perianal fistulas with human embryonic stem cell-derived mesenchymal stem cells: a canine model of human fistulizing Crohn's disease. Regenerative Medicine. 2016;**11**:33-43. DOI: 10.2217/rme.15.69

[90] Jeong J, Shin K, Lee SB, et al. Patient-tailored application for Duchenne muscular dystrophy on mdx mice based induced mesenchymal stem cells. Experimental and Molecular Pathology. 2014;**97**:253-258. DOI: 10.1016/j.yexmp.2014.08.001

[91] Liu X, Zheng L, Zhou Y, et al. BMSC transplantation aggravates inflammation, oxidative stress, and fibrosis and impairs skeletal muscle regeneration. Frontiers in Physiology. 2019;**10**:87. DOI: 10.3389/fphys.2019.00087

Chapter 6

The Impact of Payer and Reimbursement Authorities Evidence Requirements on Healthcare Solution Design for Muscular Dystrophies

Maximilian Lebmeier, Fleur Chandler, Josie Godfrey and Jonathan Dando

Abstract

For rare diseases that start early and are slowly degenerative, despite the desire to create solutions that benefit the patient, healthcare system realities can be prohibitive to generate an affordable and effective solution. The optimal care pathway for muscular dystrophy, similar to all degenerative diseases, would be a rapid and accurate diagnosis, pathophysiological confirmation and application of therapeutics that slowly replaces damaged tissue with healthy tissue, supported by adjuvant solutions that stimulate the tissue to repair and reduce inflammation and fibrosis. This would increase the lifespan and quality of life in an affordable way. For all diseases, two key stakeholders, the paying entity and the patient, fundamentally define whether revenue can be generated. Healthcare decision-making commissioners who agree to pay for the product and patient-reported outcomes jointly inform whether the intervention increases the quality of life related to existing standards of care and, therefore, if it should be paid for. This chapter explains why this has not yet happened and efforts initiated to correct this and addresses how the components and data used in this decision-making process could be updated, adapted and integrated into every stage of the development of solutions and how organisational innovation may enable the field.

Keywords: HTA, PRO, evidence generation, innovation valuation, healthcare solution development

1. Introduction

Only around 5% of the 7000 identified rare diseases have an effective treatment and this is echoed in neuromuscular conditions [1]. Recent years have witnessed a number of cancelled developments of therapeutic interventions for muscular dystrophies that were at advanced stages of development, while other interventions have been denied market authorisation, both in the US and Europe due to a lack of clinical efficacy. This means it is even more important to convince payers of the value for money of the few treatments that make it to market.

Obtaining market authorisation does not guarantee that payers will reimburse the product, that is pay for it, as growing concerns regarding the growing gap between the demand for health services and technologies and the available resources have increasingly introduced systems to assess the value for money of those products coming to market. The predominant processes for these value assessments are called health technology assessments (HTAs). Since the introduction of the National Institute for Health and Care Excellence (NICE) in 1999 in England, HTAs have spread throughout the world and now nearly every country has HTA organisations in place to help payers determine the value for money of new healthcare technologies.

These value assessments conducted by these HTA organisations consist of compiling, analysing, assessing and appraising the evidence available to show whether the health and economic benefits of a product compared to the standard of care (in the jurisdiction in question) are sufficient to justify the price, above and beyond the requirements of regulatory authorities.

There remains a lack of understanding and implementation of these considerations in clinical development without which companies will struggle to gain reimbursement.

Negative reimbursement decisions by payers hinder access to the drug substantially, if not completely. Delays in reimbursement decision-making can lead to substantial delays in a new product gaining market access. Both delays and negative decisions impact adversely on sales and consequently return of investment (ROI). Furthermore, where the evidence presented to reimbursement decision-makers bears too much uncertainty it is highly likely that the accepted price will be far below the one required by the manufacturer. Thus, investing in better data collection can support reimbursement at an acceptable price.

Given the central role played by clinical trials in generating the evidence required for HTAs, everyone involved in designing clinical trial programmes and evidence generation needs to be aware of the methods and procedures required to generate the evidence required for HTAs above and beyond the evidence requirements for regulatory approval.

This is critical for developing solutions for rare diseases, such as the muscular dystrophies, due, fundamentally, to the low number of patients, and the significant variation of disease progression and severity among the patients that makes the generation of authority stipulated convincing statistical evidence significantly more complicated [2]. There are still many treatments in late stages of clinical validation (phase II and III) and more in earlier stages of development [3] targeting as many different aspects of this multi-faceted disease as possible.

In this chapter, we present a framework for what to consider during the design of clinical trials and evidence generation alongside and beyond clinical trials for muscular dystrophies to address the evidence requirements to gain reimbursement by payers.

Concerns regarding the growing gap between demand for health services and technologies and available resources have long created the need to regulate healthcare expenditure and governments have increasingly introduced formal systems to assess the value or money of healthcare technologies coming to market [4]. Nearly every country has formal reimbursement authorities in place to help payers determine whether a health technology is worth paying for. Value assessments conducted by these authorities consist of compiling and analysing the evidence to show the health and economic benefits of a product compared to the standard of care are sufficient to justify the price desired beyond the requirements of the regulatory authorities [4].

Delays in reimbursement decision-making can lead to substantial delays in a new product gaining market access and negative reimbursement decisions by payers hinder market access substantially and thus impact adversely on sales and return on investment. Furthermore, where the evidence presented to reimbursement decision-makers bears too much uncertainty it is highly likely that the accepted price will be far below the one desired by the company. Thus, investing in better data can support reimbursement at a desired price.

Given the central role played by clinical trials in generating evidence for use in reimbursement assessments, those involved in designing clinical trials need to be aware of the evidence requirements of payers and reimbursement authorities. These differ and go beyond those of regulatory authorities.

We also explore the specifics of these issues and suggest actions that can be taken from conceptual design throughout the development of interventions that can help manufacturers unlock market access for their products. While all of the above applies to all pharmaceuticals, it is even more important in the context of muscular dystrophies and other rare disorders where data can only be generated in a small number of people as compared to more common conditions such as type 2 diabetes.

2. The patient care pathway and standard of care for the muscular dystrophies

From either a patient care and management procedure or a healthcare solution development perspective, in an ideal scenario three components are needed:

- An established and clearly defined pathophysiological assessment of the development of the disease that enables an accurate prognosis at any time point in the disease progression that a standardised diagnosis confirms;

- An overlapping and reimbursement agency-approved care pathway that defines what needs to be done at every point throughout the disease; and

- A list of the standards of care that are purchased and used throughout the care pathway.

These three components can be further complemented by population health dynamics that also integrates environmental and socio-economic components linked to patient groups that further refine best approaches.

For highly prevalent diseases, the large number of patients that are affected generates a large source of data from which statistically relevant conclusions can be drawn that inform the points above enabling healthcare practitioners to make optimised patient care decisions, while innovators can look at the pathway to identify 'pain points' for which a specific product can be created to generate a solution. For conditions such as many forms of cancer or cardiovascular diseases, this has been further augmented as global patient data collections have become integrated, thereby generating even more specific and highly tailored approaches.

Rare diseases do not and have never had the same broad evidence base as the highly prevalent diseases and that has been recognised by the key stakeholders including regulatory authorities and governments who have introduced incentives to encourage the development of new treatments for rare diseases. These stakeholders have globally networked and generated information and data resources such as the global academic network Treat NMD group (https://treat-nmd.org) focusing on all neuromuscular diseases to create a critical mass, ecosystem and hub of expertise.

Duchenne muscular dystrophy is a serious genetic disease which is life-threatening and shortens the patient's life substantially. DMD is an X-linked disorder caused by mutations in the dystrophin gene and it is the most frequent muscular dystrophy in boys affecting 1 in 3500 live births [5, 6] and 1 in 50 million girls [7]. DMD is usually diagnosed before the age of 6. The disease causes progressive and unyielding muscle weakness frequently identified in the early toddler years when the child begins to miss development motor milestones [8, 9]. Loss of ambulation occurs generally around the age of 12. Only a few DMD patients survive beyond the third decade; most die because of respiratory complications or heart failure due to cardiomyopathy [10–13].

From a clinical care perspective in DMD, because clinical care recommendations did not previously exist, the US Center for Disease control (CDC) established the DMD Care Considerations Working Group, who in 2010 published the first comprehensive DMD care considerations [12]. These were revisited and updated in 2018 to provide a complete care programme that addressed 11 key topics that occur in DMD, divided into five stages of disease [13–15]. The five recognised stages are diagnosis, early ambulatory, late ambulatory, early non-ambulatory and late non-ambulatory, and the 11 key topics include neuromuscular, rehabilitative, endocrine, gastrointestinal/nutritional, respiratory, cardiac, bone health, orthopaedic, psychosocial and transitions management. Within these publications the precise list of tests and actions that should be performed for these 11 topics at each stage are indicated. These initiatives have generated enormous amounts of benefit as proven by increased lifespans of patients and, critically, a drive to obtain even more detail about all the different characteristics of the disease and its precise progression [12, 16–19]. This has included a push to reintroduce newborn screening tools and a larger effort to understand the pathology at the earliest times of the disease, which has recently been approved by the FDA [20].

The widely held and logical argument is that the sooner the intervention is started, typically in the young child, the greater the possibility that quality of life, morbidity and length of life can be enhanced.

As the prelude to this chapter, we have analysed the approved patient care and management pathways and integrated more recent published reports on early stage assessments and longitudinal monitoring, incorporated in as much insight as possible from the most current knowledge to create a best 'what we know' about the progression of muscular dystrophies, with a bias towards Duchenne muscular dystrophy (DMD). This has been done on the basis that by analysing one muscular disease as comprehensively as possible it will complement insights from our peers for the additional muscular dystrophies.

All muscular dystrophies are genetic; DMD is X-linked and can be an inherited mutation, a spontaneous mutation or due to germline mosaicism. The onset of DMD is illustrated by a list of manifestations that serve as 'possible indicators' of the disease that then precipitates a diagnostic assessment pathway that confirms or refutes the evaluation [13].

As demonstrated in the Norwegian paediatric DMD population, if there is a family history of muscular dystrophy, then this can mean that a confirmed diagnosis is possible almost immediately (mean age at diagnosis 2.8 years with a standard deviation of 3.2 years) [21] if there is not; then indicators such as speech delay, high Creatinine Kinase or transaminases, abnormal gait or delayed motor development followed by more specific genetic tests are used to confirm diagnosis that may not occur until the child is between 3 and 6 years of age. Newborn screening for high CK is a good predictor of DMD.

Why is this important? Until recently, understanding of muscular dystrophy during the neonate phase was very limited and it was speculated that there was a 'honeymoon period' during which the disease did not develop significantly. Following the creation of the Bayley III child development assessment tool, the MDA-DMD clinical research assessed 24 children with ages ranging from 0.37 months to 2.99 years [9]. The Bayley III tool assesses children in five developmental domains: cognition, language, social–emotional, motor and adaptive behaviour. It exists in tailored forms for specific diseases. For all patients, their language and cognitive skills were lower than healthy patients, as were their fine motor skills, while the gross motor skills were more significantly impacted, implying that the large muscle groups and the core muscle groups are being affected in these patients at an early age, and it was observed that these skills declined with age. In a 1-year follow-up, declining motor function continued to be observed [22]. This work was further confirmed in a larger study involving 114 patients in which delays in gross motor development were observed [23]. Similarly in the 4D-DMD study performed comparing the healthcare records and questionnaires of 76 patients with DMD compared to 19,000 patients from the general population revealed impaired gross motor development, with first signs visible at 2–3 months of age and more evident by 24 months of age [24].

Additionally there is early fibrosis in the newborn, and the possibility there may be a cardiac involvement without overt clinical signs [25], whether there are endocrinological or respiratory issues early in development is still unclear [26]. Given the gross motor involvement, it is possible that the diaphragm maybe affected, but no respiratory analyses in very young children have been reported. The diaphragm and abdominal muscles work in tandem to stabilise the spine and trunk and enable voluntary limb movement [27].

The standard of care is to start steroid treatment and physiotherapy from the age of 3 or 4, cardiac monitoring and spirometry, measuring pulmonary function and vital capacity, from the age of 6 [13–15] and it is known that from the age of 6 onwards there is respiratory decline peaking at around 14 years of age, with a forced vital capacity (FVC) of 1 L [28] while a healthy child typically has a FVC of over 3 L. Those patients with a strong FVC have been reported to live longer [29], so we can speculate based on the outcomes from the Bayley III analysis if respiratory assessment or diaphragm thickness analysis may also be worthwhile measures at early stages of disease that can be assessed more frequently in the family practice setting, providing the equipment is available and correctly maintained [30].

How to approach this from a rehabilitative approach, especially in the neonate, given their developmental and overall regenerative capacity could be avenues to explore experimentally in animal models. It is recommended that excessive and high-impact exercise should be avoided in these patients due to the induction of muscle damage, without the normal muscle repair mechanism, thereby augmenting inflammation and fibrosis [31]. However if there is specific muscle involvement enabling a localised application of regenerative approaches combined with occupational therapy or low-intensity rehabilitation, this may provide a foundation to prevent core muscle decline, and enable other therapies to be sequentially applied. Experimentally, this has been demonstrated in traumatic muscle damage [32, 33], while in Sarcopenia low-intensity electrical stimulation has demonstrated benefits [34, 35]. Whether these approaches can be innovated and combined, while addressing the genetic aspect is an open question; however, as shown for traumatic spinal cord injuries, combination approaches can offer benefit [36].

What happens next, generally to the patient is well documented and increasingly being reported linked to the type of mutation that the patient has (nonsense, frameshift, splicing site, pseudoexon or missense). Using North Star Ambulatory Assessment (NSAA) as the outcome assessment, mild increases are observed in functionality very early and then from the age of 3 to 6.5 years the patient's ambulatory capacity increases [16] but it never reaches the age standardised healthy norm. Physical support maybe needed from the age of 8, and between the ages of 10 and 12 most patients no longer have the ability to walk, which also leads to orthopaedic-related issues (contractures in the ankles and scoliosis in 90% of patients) with associated impacts on cardiovascular and pulmonary function.

It is important to look at the specifics of each patient because of the patient variability (genetic type and likely population health-related compounding factors) and the 11 topics that are considered essential in patient care and management, as demonstrated by the studies of Phillips and Brogna [29, 37]. Despite mean assessments based upon Spirometry or 6MWT that indicate downward decline, at the individual patient level while eventually each patient's condition deteriorates, the variation between the genetic mutation (whether it is an early or late deletion, a duplication or premature stop codon) related to functionality or lung capacity indicates that there are additional compounding factors that influence pathology progression.

One trend does seem to be clear and that is when a patient's condition does deteriorate, it happens rapidly, in less than 12 months. This would suggest that a higher frequency of testing may be needed, which would for most families present a logistical problem. Therefore, patient management solutions that can be implemented either virtually as that performed in standard cardiac monitoring or in family care practices may offer innovative interim patient care and management alternatives.

Considering that every patient is typically monitored via a dedicated specialist centre, who without question perform as many of the recommended tests as possible, because no correlation has been reported between disease progression at the biometrics being assessed, there may be external factors influencing disease progression. This is not a strange phenomenon, in the instance of asthma, increased incidences of asthma are reported in lower income families, because in many cases the houses can be either mouldy or damp resulting in spores entering the child's lungs and inducing the disease [38]. It may therefore be worthwhile to integrate Population Health specialists into the ecosystem to provide additional insights, which may not generate an intervention, but will define an optimised and implementable care pathway that integrates for as many patient-specific non-disease specific variables as possible that can include broad social, socio-economic, environmental conditions as well as healthcare policies.

The cumulative outcome will hopefully be not only a globally standardised care pathway for all patients with muscular dystrophy, but also the creation of intervention and diagnostic innovations that will address reimbursement agencies' requirements and standards.

3. The evolution of reimbursement decision-making

Concerns regarding the growing gap between demand for health services and technologies and available resources have long created the need to regulate healthcare expenditure and governments have increasingly introduced formal systems to assess the value for money of healthcare technologies coming to market [4]. The predominant processes to do so are health technology assessments (HTAs) (ref).

The introduction of the National Institute for Health and Care Excellence (NICE) in 1999 in England significantly contributed to the globalisation of HTAs [39]. Nearly every country now has an HTA organisation in place to help payers determine the value of new medical interventions (**Figure 1**) [40].

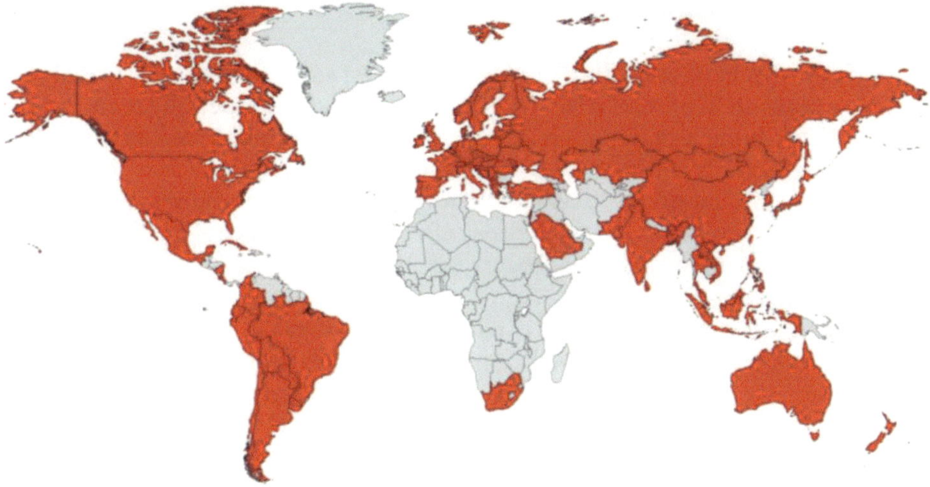

Figure 1.
Countries with formal HTA systems worldwide.

Historically, HTAs were performed after regulatory marketing authorisation had been granted. Due to the resulting gap between marketing authorisation and reimbursement, HTAs tend now to start much earlier—often in parallel with regulatory approval processes.

While there are differences between countries regarding defining the value of a new health technology, certain central requirements are common and can be addressed in clinical trials and evidence generation alongside and beyond clinical trials.

HTA is constantly evolving—the methods and processes as well the countries using it. Therefore, manufacturers developing healthcare technologies need to follow and engage with HTA developments either directly or through the use of expert consultants.

4. HTA vs regulatory requirements

Regulatory authorities around the world require manufacturers to demonstrate the risks vs. benefits and quality based on clinical and non-clinical information. Reimbursement authorities require companies to demonstrate the comparative value of their product vs. the standard of care used in their jurisdiction. To do this, they appraise a new health technology or indication in comparing a set of product attributes relating to its efficacy, safety, impact on quality of life (QoL) and functional status and pricing compared to the current standard of care.

Evidence used in HTAs for assessing the relative clinical and cost-effectiveness of new pharmaceuticals comes from a variety of sources, such as systematic literature reviews, indirect treatment comparisons and economic modelling. However, clinical trials conducted during the drug development process provide the most important source of treatment effect data for HTAs.

In recent years, some regulators including the EMA and FDA have taken steps to enable faster access to some drugs for rare conditions. For example, grant conditional authorisation to treatments such as Ataluren for DMD. This is not without controversy and HTA authorities have expressed concern that there may be insufficient evidence available for them to determine the effectiveness and value of such treatments.

5. Common HTA data needs

Traditionally, most medicines received marketing authorisation after completion of large phase III clinical trials. Increasingly, medicines, especially such with novel or breakthrough status, are receiving regulatory approval based on much smaller phase II trials and/or non-comparative 'single arm' trials.

Therefore, it is important to consider the specific evidence requirements for HTAs (i.e. core of relative clinical and cost-effectiveness evidence) much earlier in clinical development programmes, that is, when designing phase II trials as well as when designing phase III trials.

Pharmaceutical companies need to consider five critical areas when designing clinical trials to be HTA ready as well as ready for regulatory authorities:

i. Choice of comparator

ii. Measurement of clinical effectiveness

iii. Quality of life (QoL) and patient reported outcomes

iv. The collection of resource use data

v. Follow-up time of the trial

5.1 Choice of comparator

Non-comparative/single arm trials create issues when HTA decision-makers try to compare the new technology vs. the standard of care. Placebo-controlled trials result in similar issues, if the placebo arm of the trial differs substantially from clinical practice. Both result in the need of extensive indirect treatment comparisons (ITCs), thus weakening the relevance and robustness of the clinical evidence in HTAs.

We recommend, wherever possible, to use the standard of care as the comparator. This may be difficult where there is no gold standard and/or where clinical practice across and/or within countries involved in the trial varies. In such cases, we recommend consideration of the use of an active comparator based on physician choice to enable treatment comparisons relevant to HTA decision-makers in their respective jurisdictions.

5.2 Measurement of clinical effectiveness (efficacy and safety)

HTA requires outcomes to be patient relevant, and there is a growing interest in the use of patient reported outcome measures (PROMs) in clinical trials [41–43]. In some disease areas, for example cancer, it may not be possible to power a trial to capture the treatment effect on hard outcomes, such as mortality/overall survival, and surrogate endpoints are used, such as progression free survival, which is an issue for ensuring the trial results are relevant to patient outcomes. However, surrogate endpoints can be useful when a clear and robust link can be established with patient relevant outcomes. For example, as for the link between HbA1c in type 2 diabetes and cardiovascular events. However, this is only when those links have been or can be validated by studies, so that HTA decision-makers can accept them.

We recommend, where possible, to select endpoints relevant to patient outcomes (for example survival, PROMs—see more below). Where this is not possible, we recommend establishing robust links between surrogate endpoints and patient outcomes and to validate them in separate studies or with external databases.

When considering the selection of endpoints for a clinical trial, it is also important to keep in mind how the data will be used in HTAs where the new technology will be compared with other technologies used in clinical practice via an ITC. Therefore, it is important to review which endpoints have been collected in trials of most relevant comparator technologies to enable such treatment comparisons.

We recommend reviewing the endpoints used in previous trials, undertaking validation of these measures, whether the MCID is relevant and a predictor of patient outcomes and making a recommendation for consistent measures going forward to support comparisons between treatments.

However, there is non-alignment between the entities that provide market authorisation and those that perform HTAs. The FDA strongly recommends placebo-controlled trials [44], whereas the EMA suggests placebo in a two-way design study that enables a standard of care add on. With the caveat that if patients are being treated with corticosteroids, further patient stratification between the groups should be performed [45]. In both cases, a restoration of function or slowing decline is considered the main recommended endpoint, along with additional studies addressing activity levels, cardiac function and respiratory activity, while patient reported outcomes are suggested but not recommended.

Similarly, NICE in their evaluation of Idebenone, indicated that outcome measures to be considered could include pulmonary function, cardiac function, walking ability, motor function, muscle strength and HR-QOL, to assess the impact on quality of life [46].

This, however, is not reflected in the analysis of phase II and III clinical trials either performed or ongoing for muscular dystrophies. Of the 19 drugs tested in numerous phase III studies only 6 included PRO to enable a HR-QOL assessment, while of the 18 in phase II studies only 2 included PRO. One has to anticipate that because of the low number of patients in rare disease clinical trials and the importance of the impact of obtaining quality of life information to enable patients to have access to these medicines, PRO should become a standard in clinical studies, and that the PRO should be standardised throughout the field.

5.3 Quality of life (QoL) and patient reported outcomes (PROs)

HTA organisations use QoL and functional status data either for use in cost-effectiveness evaluations or as individual value attributes of additional benefit a new technology offers. A separate economic model needs to be developed (typically in Excel) to utilise input data from the clinical studies and other sources.

To support the economic value case for a new pharmaceutical, the instruments used in the trial need to allow the generation of utilities (QALYs). For utility measurement, data from generic health status measures, like the EQ-5D, tend to be preferred by HTA organisations.

For muscular dystrophies, PROs that inform changes in quality of life have been investigated to identify and tailor QoL since at least 2011 [47, 48]. The issue is that the consequences of the disease are broad and diverse, vary from patient to patient and change as a function of age. For the most juvenile patients, outcomes are dependent on parent and physician reports due to a vocabulary limitation common to all young children. To some extent, this can be replaced with the overlapping Bayley III assessment, which can assess neonate responsiveness and functionality while simultaneously evaluating if the child has developmental differences [9]. Bayley III is not a QoL indicator per se, but in the context of neonate development, the comparison between healthy and DMD patients has revealed outcomes that would suggest that this could be used for the earliest possible assessment. It is essential to read this publication for the indicated outcomes for functional expectation of healthy neonates and how this compares to patients with muscular dystrophy, because of the emphasis that regulatory bodies give to functional gains.

Following this, PROs are obtained routinely using the Paediatric Outcomes Data Collection Instrument (PODCI), SF-36 Health survey [41] and Neuromuscular module and Generic Core Scales of the PedsQL, which are also suggested by the EMA [45]. However, measuring QoL becomes significantly more complex as the patient grows. It has been reported that QoL outcomes using the PedsQL become unreliable as the patient ages [47], at least in the context of restoration of function, as defined by regulatory bodies versus increases in quality of life. The insinuation is that a restoration in function does not necessarily correlate to an increase in quality of life, which reinforces the concept that selected population health-related or additional pathophysiological measurements may need to be integrated into the appraisal as a third axis.

Additional research has been performed utilising the WHO ICF-CY [19, 49, 50], while the most comprehensive research on identifying, designing and optimising PRO specific for the muscular dystrophies has been reported from ScHARR [41–43] that forms a core part of the Project HERCULES initiative, a project led by the patient organisation Duchenne UK, aimed towards creating a suite of disease level HTA evidence including QoL assessment for DMD. The emphasis is that the QoL questionnaire needs to retain core expectations while also expanding the readouts as a function of neurological gain as the patient matures and can expand their expressiveness.

In muscular dystrophies, Project HERCULES (see below) is developing an optimised Duchenne muscular dystrophy (DMD)-specific instrument to create a preference-based measure to meet the needs of HTA.

Besides their use in cost-effectiveness evaluations, the use of generic and condition-specific instruments will generate data to inform HTA decision-makers' assessments of the additional benefit of the new technology compared to the standard of care as individual value attributes.

QoL and functional status data should be collected at baseline and throughout the trial and follow-up period.

We recommend collecting QoL and functional status data using generic health status measures that allow the generation of utilities, as well as including a condition-specific instrument. In selecting which PROMs to choose, it is important to review the trials of the most relevant comparators to enable better comparison between technologies during HTAs.

5.4 The collection of resource use data

This includes hospitalisations, outpatient/GP appointments and tests/investigations to inform the cost-effectiveness analysis. There is no universally recognised method for economic data collection in clinical trials and a variety of techniques are used. The methods and instruments used should reflect the health condition to new technology addresses. The researcher planning the trial should again review the trials of the most relevant comparators to identify potential methods and instruments.

Resource use data should be collected at baseline and throughout the trial and follow-up period. However, resource use data collection from a multinational clinical trial should be performed with caution due to the concerns over the generalisability of the data for country-specific HTA submissions. Hence, there is a key role for local validation of resource use estimates from a trial and/or observational data collection. Additional Burden of Illness studies should be undertaken alongside trials to show real-world evidence.

5.5 Follow-up time of the trial

Studies should have an appropriately long enough follow-up time to enable the collection of consistent, sufficient and robust data relevant to HTA decision-makers. Minimising uncertainty about clinical effectiveness may be a particular challenge for life-long progressive conditions with limited data such as muscular dystrophies and there is no fixed time period favoured by HTA bodies.

In addition, a plan detailing how and when individual endpoints will be collected is essential. This should include the frequency, methods, sources and time horizon within the data. Besides the data collection plan, the researcher planning the trial should also consider the development of a specific health economics/HTA statistical analyses plan (SAP) covering such aspects as to how PROM and resource use data will be analysed for HTA and use in economic models. This would complement the regular clinical study SAP.

6. HTA scientific advice

Some HTA bodies, for example NICE, offer HTA-specific scientific advice to developers of health technologies to help them develop evidence required for HTAs [51]. Also, the EMA and EUNetHTA (EU body responsible for co-ordinating HTA methods and policies in Europe) offer a joint scientific advice programme to companies with HTA organisations involved.

All of those processes come with varying requirements for preparation and company input and varying levels of opportunities for engagement with the involved parties.

7. Unofficial procedures

1. Advisory board meetings with health economists with clinical trial experience for selected key territories, HTA experts and clinicians to review and input into clinical trials.

2. One-to-one meetings with payer/HTA experts to review and gain input for clinical trial programmes from specific experts for specific regions and/or countries.

3. Working with specialist health economics consultants with clinical trial, HTA scientific advice and HTA experience to review plans, gain input into clinical trials, to develop whole HTA scientific advice programme tailored to the individual company requirements and to provide wider market access and HTA advice also supporting and/or conducting individual projects.

4. Patient and family input is crucial to fully understand the impact of the disease, on health, quality of life, socially and financially as well as any practical considerations relating to the feasibility of the trial design.

For all of the above, we recommend working with health economists with clinical trial and HTA experience to review plans, gain input into clinical trials, to develop whole HTA scientific advice programme tailored to the individual company requirements and to provide wider market access and HTA advice also supporting and/or conducting individual projects. This can also include the consultants helping the company to navigate the official procedures.

8. Evidence generation alongside and beyond clinical trials

Beyond clinical evidence generation, developers of healthcare technologies need to develop a set of HTA value propositions covering the impact their technology will have on the unmet need, its comparative effectiveness demonstration (planned and expected and/or based on potentially available data), patient reported outcomes (including quality of life), cost-effectiveness, and resource use, costs and budget impact as well as covering a PICO (Patient, Intervention, Comparator and Outcomes) statement.

Companies need to conduct early HTA-specific gap analyses and HTA feasibility assessments to identify gaps in their own as well as their comparator's evidence base to allow for sufficient time to fill those through evidence generation within, alongside and beyond clinical trials. With this, it is also important to remember that HTA preparations need to start early with HTA input into phase II clinical trial planning and designing at the very latest and from there on being a constant and equal (to regulatory) part of any development as getting reimbursement is equally important as getting a marketing authorisation.

9. Other considerations

Companies need to conduct early economic modelling and payer research to inform their pricing strategy reflecting their evidence base. Technologies that are too expensive and do not have a significant benefit over existing alternatives are unlikely to be approved. The key driver of cost in many economic evaluations submitted to HTA organisations is the price of the technology. Where the list price is too high for the technology to be approved for reimbursement, companies can provide discounts and/or other commercial arrangements to reduce the cost to an approvable level. There are also instances when a new technology may be additive to existing standards of care. Where this care is already expensive, it is possible for a new treatment to not be cost-effective even at zero cost [52].

In other instances, it is not the list price of the technology but the uncertainty of the submitted benefits driving the need for a discount and/or commercial arrangement. In HTAs evidence uncertainty is critical and higher the uncertainty the lower the acceptable price will be. Therefore, investing in better data and filling evidence gaps as early as possible can support a better price and avoid the need for a discount and/or commercial requirement.

Economic modelling can help a company to identify the potential need for a discount or commercial arrangement and where they are required the potential magnitude required.

Beyond evidence generation and pricing, manufacturers should follow and engage with HTA developments, follow comparator HTAs to inform their own HTA preparations and be open, transparent, collaborative and realistic when engaging with HTA authorities.

Support is available to companies throughout the whole process from early development through to the conclusion of individual HTAs from official bodies, like HTA organisations, as well as from experienced HTA expert consultants. Companies should make use of the support available to them.

Furthermore, stakeholders from different backgrounds involved in addressing challenges in healthcare are increasingly working together cross functionally and globally. Developers of treatments for muscular dystrophies should also consider such approaches where they are not already happening. One outstanding example of such a collaboration in muscular dystrophies is Project HERCULES [53, 54].

10. Project HERCULES

In the field of Duchenne muscular dystrophy (DMD), one of the most common and severe forms of muscular dystrophy, Duchenne UK set up Project HERCULES (HEalth Research Collaboration United in Leading Evidence Synthesis) to develop tools and evidence to support HTA for new treatments for DMD [53–55].

Many pharmaceutical companies are developing potential treatments for DMD and are working individually to develop their approach to HTA. The variety of methods in use and the difficulties of generating data can lead to delays in introducing new treatments and inconsistent decision-making.

Duchenne UK invited pharmaceutical companies with a DMD product in development to a training day in February 2017 to explore modelling and HTA in DMD. This led to the establishment of Project HERCULES, a collaborative global project bringing together patient organisations, clinicians, academics, nine active pharmaceutical companies, HTA agencies and other advisors.

Project HERCULES has generated a set of disease-level evidence and tools including a natural history model, burden of disease data, a de novo DMD-specific quality of life metric, and a core economic model. These individual workstreams have been developed in parallel through an iterative process enabling evidence generated for one work stream to inform the others. This iterative approach ensured that input from clinicians, patients and carers and other experts was used for multiple purposes minimising the demands on stakeholders.

The leadership of a patient organisation enabled access to data sources and expertise that may be inaccessible for individual or industry researchers. The patient organisation was also able to recruit patients and parents to participate in the research through the use of social media and offline networks. There have been clear efficiencies for manufacturers in being able to access evidence and expertise and a greatly reduced cost compared to developing these evidence and tools in isolation.

The collaborative approach taken by Project HERCULES was not without challenges. Researchers often needed to learn to explain complex concepts in accessible language to ensure patients and lay members could effectively contribute. Balancing the input from patients and families with clinical, industry and HTA experts has also been challenging. Project HERCULES selected researchers in part by their readiness to work collaboratively with stakeholders ensuring that they were working closely with the other research teams and actively listening and responding to all the information obtained, and not simply seeking confirmation for what they expected to find.

Despite the challenges, Project HERCULES has consistently taken a collaborative approach that has had a clear impact on each workstream:

- Enabling researchers to test assumptions against lived experience and develop their own understanding of the condition and care pathway

- Identification of meaningful disease stages including the previously overlooked transfer state between the traditional stages of late ambulatory and early non-ambulatory. Patient and parents told researchers about the importance of being able to weight bear for a period following the loss of ambulation. This state has been incorporated into the natural history model, which informs the other work streams.

- Development of a bespoke Quality of Life preference based measure that better reflects the lived experiences of those with DMD as well as the views of clinicians and other experts.

- An economic model that builds on the actual experience of clinicians, patients and families

- A burden of illness study focusing on what is most important to clinicians, patients and families.

11. Impact on investment and return on investment

In healthcare, and particularly therapeutic intervention, development takes a long time, typically over 14 years [56, 57], and is costly (up to $2.6 billion, [58]), which means that significant risk has to be carried for a long duration before knowing if the product was worth the investment. However, in the context of rare diseases, the scenario is significantly different. Whereas the development up to launch of a medicine for a very common condition may cost $2.6 Billion, for the muscular dystrophies the value might be closer to $400 Million. The number of patients involved in the trials are significantly lower, the duration of the trials shorter and upon market release, an extensive sales force is not necessary, as patients are typically referred to centres of excellence [59–61], and clinicians who focus on treating patients with rare diseases are typically well versed in developments in the field, while patients associations perform stellar work in communicating with patients and their supporters what is happening [7, 62–68]. As explained above, achieving a marketing authorisation does not guarantee reimbursement that companies need to achieve before they can realise uptake and sales.

This leads us to two questions: (a) what impact integrating HTA requirements in clinical trial design has on investment decision-making, and (b) what impact it has on return on investment.

To answer the first question, we need to look at how pharmaceutical investment decisions are informed.

The decision to invest in the creation of a medical product, as for all other businesses, hinges on the definition of the market size, the terminal market value. The terminal market value is then reverse calculated to the potential present value by integrating in phase specific costs, risks and probabilities of success to give a net present value (NPV). If the NPV is positive, then the innovation is considered worthwhile to invest in, whereas if it is negative, the rule of thumb is to not invest.

NPV calculations are only as good as the data used to generate them, and both accurate and comprehensive values ideally should be used, based on real market dynamic, the latest clinical success rates and considering the latest reimbursement approaches (such as HTAs). Thus, designing clinical trials that are more likely to result in better data and addressing HTA evidence requirements improve NPV calculations and thus optimise investment decision-making [69]. However, it is important to state that there is the possibility that market authorisation agencies and reimbursement bodies may not accept clinical data from other jurisdictions due to different standards and regulations. Therefore, while NPV outputs are additive, the developer may need to assess if different clinical trials need to be performed in different locations and if and how the data can be used within a comprehensive evidence dossier that can be submitted to as many different agencies as possible.

The answer to the second question is that investing in better evidence generation will lead to higher chances of gaining desired reimbursement at the desired price, thus unlocking market access and sales potential early, thus having a positive impact on ROI. For the rare diseases, accounting for post-marketing surveillance, manufacturing and general admin costs, to reach a balance of zero, the product will need to generate at least $1 Billion in life time sales; to enable the innovators to sustain and expand their pipeline, generating additional new interventions for other rare diseases, life time sales between $2 Billion and $8 Billion would be required. Based on marketing authorisation restrictions on recently approved DMD interventions, that are based upon the differing forms of dystrophinopathies, this revenue level would need to be generated from generating a beneficial effect (clinical effectiveness and cost effectiveness) for 10% of the muscular dystrophy population, who would likely need to administer the solution every year for the rest of their life, that could be an additional 25 years based on the increased standards of care. This combined information is then used to define the agreed price of the solution with the reimbursement agency, within the specifics of the healthcare system and marketplace in each different geography (this can be an entire country or a region within a country).

Governments have tried to be flexible to account for the market risks, policy changes have been implemented, such as the orphan drug definition in the EU. Because of the potentially low revenue potential, investing in solutions for rare diseases carries a higher risk, as costs cannot be recovered, therefore acts that provide market exclusivity for 12 years for paediatric diseases, in competition with 'similar competitive products'. Additionally, to facilitate R&D in healthcare, most countries offer R&D tax credits, independent of the source of the R&D funding, and using a very broad definition of what constitutes a R&D cost to stimulate such endeavours. These credits can be used to offset taxes on profit, providing the entity reinvests the revenue.

Conceptually for a paediatric rare disease, the rule may need to be revisited to reconsider what is the definition of a similar product to provide clarity to innovators. Arguably it is any intervention that offers disease correction, which can be a very broad definition or is it based upon similar mechanisms of action; ideally innovators would need this point clarified to enable better clinical trial design. This is reflected in the clinical trials that are ongoing and appear to be following the conceptual design associated with major diseases, that is an 'all or nothing' response based upon the intervention being assessed.

Given that the disease takes years to manifest itself, and varies significantly from patient to patient as seen in other progressive degenerative diseases or traumatic injuries with inconsistent and differing measurements, it is more likely that a spectrum of concepts and solutions need to be integrated together as function of the patient and the tissue damage at that specific stage within the complete disease progression to provide beneficial outcomes; this is likely going to include standard chemical entity interventions, anti-inflammatories and physiotherapy and potentially stem cells, biomaterials, genetic correction, tailored and designed as a comprehensive intervention solution tailored to the patient and their population health status.

12. Conclusions

In summary, we would like to emphasise that for a product to be able to get a positive HTA recommendation leading to reimbursement by payers, manufacturers need to carefully consider the evidence needs of HTA authorities when planning clinical trials and evidence generation programmes.

For each new product, this should start early, that is when planning phase II trials, and continue throughout the clinical development process in order to optimise the chances of gaining reimbursement and consequently return of investment.

Beyond evidence generation and pricing companies follow and engage with HTA developments, follow comparator HTAs to inform their own HTA preparations and be open, transparent, collaborative and realistic when engaging with HTA authorities.

Support is available to manufacturers throughout the whole process from early development through to the conclusion of individual HTAs from official bodies, like HTA organisations, as well as from experienced HTA expert consultants. Additionally, innovative initiatives, such as Project HERCULES, are existing to support developers but also serve as examples of what is possible and can be done beyond existing support structures and options. Manufacturers should make use of the support available to them.

Furthermore, addressing the evidence requirements of payers and HTA organisations in clinical trials and other evidence generation can lead to improved investment decision-making and have a positive impact on ROI.

It is also important to emphasise that developers of healthcare technologies need to address the evidence needs of reimbursement decision-makers early and throughout the development process in order to optimise their chances of gaining market access at a desired price unlocking ROI. To obtain and support this outcome, there may need to be a reconfiguration of the muscular dystrophy R&D ecosystem. A large amount of fundamental research has been and is still performed in the muscular dystrophies, mostly paid by charities such as MDA, Telethon, Duchenne and AFM, to name only a few. In no way does the volume of research and funding for muscular dystrophy compare to the major diseases.

For the major diseases, the years of highly funded fundamental research has resulted in outcomes that have translated to the clinic for the benefit of patients that is founded upon a significant amount of independently validated and reproduced data. Naturally, at the public funding level, policy is therefore biased towards encouraging fundamental research to have a translatable dimension to justify to the taxpayer the expense.

Rare disease researchers have not had a large knowledge resource but find themselves in the position that they need to accelerate their translatable research, due to patient need, without the same foundation of knowledge to rely upon. This is not going to change; however, different approaches to managing the knowledge that is generated from the limited financial support that is given to fundamental research in the muscular dystrophies would be beneficial for this field, other muscular diseases and the rare diseases field as a whole. But the barriers to progression are compounded by additional characteristics that are common to all other diseases and the culture of R&D and others that are unique to the field of muscular dystrophy.

One significant issue in knowledge generation in the muscular dystrophies is the genotypic diversity within each type that often prevents statistically relevant insights being obtained that can be leveraged into intervention development. This is because to obtain some level of relevant data the work has to be performed in an animal model that corresponds to the specific disease genotype. This means creating the model (often a mouse) through transgenic modification, and after stabilising the model, assessing if the genotypic change generates a disease phenotype that corresponds to the human form of disease. On the proviso that a comprehensive understanding of the disease progression and phenotype is understood in the human.

Pre-clinical modelling is used to generate data that show a corrective effect, levels of toxicity, intervention metabolism and potential dosing. After generation of the comprehensive dossier for review, a positive ethical review board will then permit a phase I testing of the drug in humans. The aim is to define if the considered therapeutic dose is toxic to a healthy human. If it is confirmed that the therapeutic does not harm a human, it is then approved to test in a small population of patients if in addition to not harming the patient it confers some level of corrective effect (phase IIa). If positive, the study can be expanded to more patients (phase IIb). Positive data from this phase enable the larger scale phase III, efficacy study on large patient populations. For diabetes and CVD, the available patient population for recruitment is huge.

For muscular dystrophies it is not; this means that a substantial amount of evidence has to be generated from between 30 to 250 patients, if they correspond to the inclusion/exclusion criteria of the trial, which typically includes not taking other experimental interventions. Independent of whether a disease is rare or frequent, this is not possible. It would be impossible and likely rejected by market authorisation bodies if this approach was taken for a highly prevalent disease as an evidence collection method. Policy changes have occurred focusing on rare diseases to be more flexible on effect and patient numbers, but clinical trial design still hinges on an 'all or nothing' therapeutic effect from a single intervention. This does not correspond to the complexity of muscle tissue, the diversity between patients, the impact of comorbidities and the regenerative characteristics of muscle.

For fundamental researchers, specifically those in academia who perform most of the fundamental research operate in a 'publish or perish' professional environment. The nature of fundamental R&D is that >90% of the data generated, at first glance, is a negative result, and the space limitations in articles accepted for publication means that even very limited positive results are shown. A negative result being defined as an outcome that does not correspond to enabling a chosen question to be answered, it does not mean the data are useless or invaluable.

With such limited resources, financially, biologically and clinically, but with such a clear patient need, the field needs to reconsider how it best leverages its data, especially as there are not a high number of researchers active in muscular dystrophy, in comparison to cancer or cardiovascular diseases.

This could be resolved through a 'research data' database that can be accessed by all accredited researchers to enable searching other historical data from other sources to look for concepts that did not work to prevent wasteful repetition, or to look at the unpublished data with a new perspective to enable a different insight. This also needs to happen with clinical data, from those patients in trials to those having their disease history mapped, albeit with a greater ethical oversight. There are nearly 13,000 patients presently in global clinical trials for Limb Girdle, Beckers and Duchenne muscular dystrophy who will be generating what may first appear to be non-relevant data related to the defined outcomes, but it is very likely that in the context of age, disease progression, biometrics, comorbidity status, mental health status, population health characteristics as well as response to intervention, these data are going to massively inform the field and globally standardised clinical care pathways and patient biometric measurements.

Author details

Maximilian Lebmeier[1,2], Fleur Chandler[3], Josie Godfrey[4] and Jonathan Dando[2,5]*

1 Athena Market Access Solutions Ltd, UK

2 Aestimo Ltd, Ireland

3 Duchenne UK, UK

4 JG Zebra Consulting Ltd, UK

5 Echino Ltd, UK

*Address all correspondence to: jdando@aestimo.ie

References

[1] Kaufmann P, Pariser AR, Austin C. From scientific discovery to treatments for rare diseases—The view from the National Center for Advancing Translational Sciences—Office of Rare Diseases Research. Orphanet Journal of Rare Diseases. 2018;**13**:196. DOI: 10.1186/s13023-018-0936-x

[2] Dando J. "What did Maxwell's equations really have to do with Edison's invention?": Addressing the complexity of developing clinical interventions for skeletal muscle disease. Current Topics in Developmental Biology. 2018;**126**: 1-22. DOI: 10.1016/bs.ctdb.2017.09.001. [Epub: 23 October 2017]

[3] Duchenne Drug Development Pipeline. Parent Project Muscular Dystrophy. 2019. Available from: https://www.parentprojectmd.org/duchenne-drug-development-pipeline/ [Accessed: 05 January 2020]

[4] Lebmeier M, Tolley K. Designing clinical trials to support pharmaceutical reimbursement. Journal for Clinical Studies. 2019;**11**(4)

[5] Katirji B, Kaminski HJ, Ruff RL, editors. Neuromuscular Disorders in Clinical Practice [Internet]. 2nd ed. New York: Springer-Verlag; 2014. Available from: https://www.springer.com/us/book/9781461465669 [Accessed: 30 January 2020]

[6] Mendell JR, Rodino-Klapac LR, Sahenk Z, Roush K, Bird L, Lowes LP, et al. Eteplirsen for the treatment of Duchenne muscular dystrophy. Annals of Neurology. 2013;**74**(5):637-647

[7] Duchenne UK. Available from: https://www.duchenneuk.org [Accessed: 05 January 2020]

[8] Henricson EK, Abresch RT, Cnaan A, Hu F, Duong T, Arrieta A, et al. The Cooperative International Neuromuscular Research Group Duchenne natural history study: Glucocorticoid treatment preserves clinically meaningful functional milestones and reduces rate of disease progression as measured by manual muscle testing and other commonly used clinical trial outcome measures. Muscle & Nerve. 2013;**48**(1):55-67

[9] Connolly AM,Florence JM, Craddock MM, Malkus EC, Schierbecker JR, Siener CA, et al. Motor and cognitive assessment of infants and young boys with Duchenne muscular dystrophy: Results from the Muscular Dystrophy Association DMD Clinical Research Network. Neuromuscular Disorders. 2013;**23**(7):529-539

[10] Ricotti V, Selby V, Ridout D, Domingos J, Decostre V, Mayhew A, et al. Respiratory and upper limb function as outcome measures in ambulant and non-ambulant subjects with Duchenne muscular dystrophy: A prospective multicentre study. Neuromuscular Disorders. 2019;**29**(4):261-268

[11] Van Ruiten H, Bushby K, Guglieri M. State-of-the-art advances in Duchenne muscular dystrophy. European Medical Journal. 2017;**1**:90-99

[12] Bushby K, Finkel R, Birnkrant DJ, Case LE, Clemens PR, Cripe L, et al. Diagnosis and management of Duchenne muscular dystrophy, part 1: Diagnosis, and pharmacological and psychosocial management. Lancet Neurology. 2010;**9**(1):77-93

[13] Birnkrant DJ, Bushby K, Bann CM, Apkon SD, Blackwell A, Brumbaugh D, et al. Diagnosis and management of Duchenne muscular dystrophy, part 1: Diagnosis, and neuromuscular, rehabilitation, endocrine, and gastrointestinal and nutritional management. Lancet Neurology. 2018;**17**(3):251-267

[14] Birnkrant DJ, Bushby K, Bann CM, et al. Diagnosis and management of Duchenne muscular dystrophy, part 2: Respiratory, cardiac, bone health, and orthopaedic management. Lancet Neurology. 2018;**17**(4):347-361. DOI: 10.1016/S1474-4422(18)30025-5

[15] Birnkrant DJ, Bushby K, Bann CM, et al. Diagnosis and management of Duchenne muscular dystrophy, part 3: Primary care, emergency management, psychosocial care, and transitions of care across the lifespan. Lancet Neurology. 2018;**17**(5):445-455. DOI: 10.1016/S1474-4422(18)30026-7

[16] Coratti G, Brogna C, Norcia G, Ricotti V, Abbott L, D'Amico A, et al. Longitudinal natural history in young boys with Duchenne muscular dystrophy. Neuromuscular Disorders. 2019 Nov;**29**(11):857-862. DOI: 10.1016/j.nmd.2019.09.010. [Epub: 26 September 2019]

[17] McDonald CM, Gordish-Dressman H, Henricson EK, Duong T, Joyce NC, Jhawar S, et al. Longitudinal pulmonary function testing outcome measures in Duchenne muscular dystrophy: Long-term natural history with and without glucocorticoids. Neuromuscular Disorders. 2018;**28**(11):897-909. DOI: 10.1016/j.nmd.2018.07.004. [Epub: 29 August 2018]

[18] Lerario A, Bonfiglio S, Sormani M, et al. Quantitative muscle strength assessment in duchenne muscular dystrophy: Longitudinal study and correlation with functional measures. BMC Neurology. 2012;**12**:91. DOI: 10.1186/1471-2377-12-91

[19] Messina S, Vita GL, Sframeli M, et al. Health-related quality of life and functional changes in DMD: A 12-month longitudinal cohort study. Neuromuscular Disorders. 2016;**26**(3):189-196. DOI: 10.1016/j.nmd.2016.01.003

[20] Bigica A. FDA Authorizes First Duchenne Muscular Dystrophy Newborn Screening Test. 2019. Available from: https://www.neurologylive.com/clinical-focus/fda-authorizes-first-duchenne-muscular-dystrophy-newborn-screening-test [Accessed: 05 January 2020]

[21] Annexstad EJ, Fagerheim T, Holm I, Rasmussen M. Molecular and clinical characteristics of a national cohort of paediatric Duchenne muscular dystrophy patients in Norway. Journal of Neuromuscular Diseases. 2019;**6**:349-359

[22] Connolly AM, Florence JM, Cradock MM, et al. One year outcome of boys with Duchenne muscular dystrophy using the Bayley-III scales of infant and toddler development. Pediatric Neurology. 2014;**50**(6):557-563. DOI: 10.1016/j.pediatrneurol.2014.02.006

[23] Miller N, Alfano L, Iammarino M, Dugan M, Moore-Clingenpeel M, Tsao C-Y, et al. Early signs of gross motor delay in very young boys with Duchenne muscular dystrophy (P1.6-068). Neurology. 2019;**92**(15 Supplement) P1.6-068.

[24] Van Dommelen P, Van Dijk O, De Wilde JA, Verkerk PH. Developmental delay in Duchenne Muscular Dystrophy: A case-control study of a Dutch population. Available from: https://repository.tudelft.nl/view/tno/uuid%3A1d0e1efd-5fad-4d06-b14a-d12dad417979 [Accessed: 05 January 2020]

[25] Case LE, Apkon SD, Eagle M, Gulyas A, Juel L, Matthews D, et al. Rehabilitation management of the patient with Duchenne muscular dystrophy. Pediatrics. 2018;**142**(Supplement 2):S17-S33. DOI: 10.1542/peds.2018-0333D

[26] LoMauro A, D'Angelo MG, Aliverti A. Assessment and management

of respiratory function in patients with Duchenne muscular dystrophy: Current and emerging options. Therapeutics and Clinical Risk Management. 2015;**11**:1475-1488. DOI: 10.2147/TCRM.S55889

[27] Kolar P, Sulc J, Kyncl M, Sanda J, Neuwirth J, Bokarius AV, et al. Stabilizing function of the diaphragm: Dynamic MRI and synchronized spirometric assessment. *Journal of Applied Physiology*. 2010;**109**:1064-1071

[28] Khirani S, Ramirez A, Aubertin G, Boulé M, Chemouny C, Forin V, et al. Respiratory muscle decline in Duchenne muscular dystrophy. Pediatric Pulmonology. 2014;**49**(5):473-481

[29] Phillips MF, Quinlivan RC, Edwards RH, Calverley PM. Changes in spirometry over time as a prognostic marker in patients with Duchenne musculardystrophy. American Journal of Respiratory and Critical Care Medicine. 2001;**164**(12):2191-2194

[30] Hegewald MJ, Gallo HM, Wilson EL. Accuracy and quality of spirometry in primary care offices. Annals of the American Thoracic Society. 2016;**13**(12):2119-2124

[31] Ansved T. Muscular dystrophies: Influence of physical conditioning on the disease evolution. Current Opinion in Clinical Nutrition and Metabolic Care. 2003;**6**(4):435-439

[32] Fuoco C, Salvatori ML, Biondo A, et al. Injectable polyethylene glycol-fibrinogen hydrogel adjuvant improves survival and differentiation of transplanted mesoangioblasts in acute and chronic skeletal-muscle degeneration. Skeletal Muscle. 2012;**2**(1):24. DOI: 10.1186/2044-5040-2-24

[33] Armstrong JPK, Puetzer JL, Serio A, et al. Engineering anisotropic muscle tissue using acoustic cell patterning. Advanced Materials. 2018;**30**(43):e1802649. DOI: 10.1002/adma.201802649

[34] Kern H, Barberi L, Löfler S, et al. Electrical stimulation counteracts muscle decline in seniors. Frontiers in Aging Neuroscience. 2014;**6**:189. DOI: 10.3389/fnagi.2014.00189

[35] Zampieri S, Mosole S, Löfler S, et al. Physical exercise in aging: Nine weeks of leg press or electrical stimulation training in 70 years old sedentary elderly people. European Journal of Translational Myology. 2015;**25**(4):237-242. DOI: 10.4081/ejtm.2015.5374

[36] Cristante AF, de Barros Filho TEP, Marcon RM, Letaif OB, da Rocha ID. Therapeutic approaches for spinal cord injury. Clinics. 2012;**67**(10):1219-1224. DOI: 10.6061/clinics/2012(10)16

[37] Brogna C, Coratti G, Pane M, et al. Long-term natural history data in Duchenne muscular dystrophy ambulant patients with mutations amenable to skip exons 44, 45, 51 and 53 [published correction appears in PLoS One. 2019 Jul 31;14(7):e0220714]. PLoS One. 2019;**14**(6):e0218683. DOI: 10.1371/journal.pone.0218683

[38] Pacheco CM, Ciaccio CE, Nazir N, et al. Homes of low-income minority families with asthmatic children have increased condition issues. Allergy and Asthma Proceedings. 2014;**35**(6):467-474. DOI: 10.2500/aap.2014.35.3792. Available from: https://www.ncbi.nlm.nih.gov/pmc/articles/PMC4210655/

[39] Drummond ME et al. Methods for the Economic Evaluation of Health Care Programmes. 3rd ed. Oxford University Press; 2005. Available from: https://www.ncbi.nlm.nih.gov/pmc/articles/PMC4210655/

[40] ISPOR HEOR Resources. 2020. Available from: https://www.ispor.org/heor-resources [Accessed: 05 January 2020]

[41] Uttley L, Carlton J, Woods HB, Brazier J. A review of quality of life themes in Duchenne muscular dystrophy for patients and carers. Health and Quality of Life Outcomes. 2018;**16**:237

[42] Powell PA, Carlton J, Rowen D, et al. Producing a preference-based quality of life measure for people with Duchenne muscular dystrophy: A mixed-methods study protocol. BMJ Open. 2019;**9**:e023685. DOI: 10.1136/bmjopen-2018-023685. Available from: https://www.ncbi.nlm.nih.gov/pmc/articles/PMC4210655/

[43] Powell P, Carlton J, Woods H, et al. Patient reported outcome measures of quality of life in Duchenne muscular dystrophy (DMD): A systematic review of content and structural validity using COSMIN. Report. ScHARR HEDS Discussion Papers. School of Health and Related Research, University of Sheffield; 2019

[44] Duchenne Muscular Dystrophy and Related Dystrophinopathies: Developing Drugs for Treatment Guidance for Industry. U.S. Department of Health and Human Services, Food and Drug Administration, Center for Drug Evaluation and Research (CDER), Center for Biologics Evaluation and Research (CBER); 2018 Clinical/Medical. Available from: https://www.fda.gov/media/92233/download [Accessed: 05 January 2020]

[45] Guideline on the clinical investigation of medicinal products for the treatment of Duchenne and Becker muscular dystrophy. 1 EMA/CHMP/236981/2011, Corr. 1 Committee for Medicinal Products for Human Use (CHMP). 2015. Available from: https://www.ema.europa.eu/en/documents/scientific-guideline/guideline-clinical-investigation-medicinal-products-treatment-duchenne-becker-muscular-dystrophy_en.pdf [Accessed: 05 January 2020]

[46] National Institute for Health and Care Excellence. Proposed Health Technology Appraisal Idebenone for Treating Duchenne Muscular Dystrophy Draft Scope (Pre-Referral) NICE 2017. Available from: https://www.nice.org.uk/guidance/gid-ta10310/ documents/draft-scope-pre-referral [Accessed: 05 January 2020]

[47] Grootenhuis MA, De Boone J, Van der Kooi AJ. Living with muscular dystrophy: Health related quality of life consequences for children and adults. Health and Quality of Life Outcomes. 2007;**5**(1):1

[48] Baiardini I et al. Quality of life in Duchenne muscular dystrophy: The subjective impact on children and parents. Journal of Child Neurology. 2011;**26**(6):707-713

[49] International classification of functioning, disability and health: children & youth version: ICF-CY. Available from: https://apps.who.int/iris/bitstream/handle/10665/43737/?sequence=1 [Accessed: 05 January 2020]

[50] Bendixen et al. Participation and quality of life in children with Duchenne muscular dystrophy using the International Classification of Functioning, Disability, and Health. Health and Quality of Life Outcomes. 2012;**10**:43

[51] NICE Scientific Advice. Available from: https://www.nice.org.uk/about/what-we-do/life-sciences/scientific-advice [Accessed: 26 January 2020]

[52] Assessing Technologies that are not Cost-Effective at a Zero Price. 2020. Available from: http://nicedsu.

org.uk/methods-development/not-cost-effective-at-0/

[53] Project Hercules. Available from: https://hercules.duchenneuk.org/ [Accessed: 26 January 2020]

[54] Project Hercules 2. Available from: https://hercules.duchenneuk.org/about-project-hercules/ [Accessed: 26 January 2020]

[55] NHS—Muscular Dystrophy. Available from: https://www.nhs.uk/conditions/muscular-dystrophy/ [Accessed: 26 January 2020]

[56] FDA. The Drug Development and Approval Process. 2016. Available from: http://www.fdareview.org/03_drug_development.php [Accessed: 05 January 2020]

[57] Stewart JJ, Allison PN, Johnson RS. Putting a price on biotechnology. Nature Biotechnology Bioentrepreneur. 2018. DOI: 10.1038/nbt0901-813. Available from: https://www.nature.com/bioent/2003/030101/full/nbt0901-813.html

[58] DiMasi JA, Grabowski HG, Hansen RW. Innovation in the pharmaceutical industry: New estimates of R&D costs. Journal of Health Economics. 2016;**47**:20-33

[59] Neuromusclar Centres of Excellence Awards, Muscular Dystrophy UK. Available from: https://www.musculardystrophyuk.org/your-stories/neuromuscular-centres-of-excellence/ [Accessed: 05 January 2020]

[60] Parent Project Certified Care Centers. Available from: https://www.parentprojectmd.org/care/find-a-certified-duchenne-care-center/ [Accessed: 05 January 2020]

[61] MDA Care Centers. Available from: https://www.mda.org/care/mda-care-centers [Accessed: 05 January 2020]

[62] Muscular Dystrophy Association. Available from: https://www.mda.org/about-mda [Accessed: 05 January 2020]

[63] Parent Project. Available from: https://www.parentprojectmd.org [Accessed: 05 January 2020]

[64] Action Duchenne. Available from: https://www.actionduchenne.org/about-us/ [Accessed: 05 January 2020]

[65] CureCMD. Available from: https://www.curecmd.org/mission-history [Accessed: 05 January 2020]

[66] LGMD2i. Available from: https://www.lgmd2ifund.org [Accessed: 05 January 2020]

[67] Treat NMD. Available from: https://treat-nmd.org/about-the-treat-nmd-network/ [Accessed: 05 January 2020]

[68] AFM. Available from: http://www.afm-telethon.com/about-afm/missions.html [Accessed: 05 January 2020]

[69] Dando J, Lebmeier M. A novel valuation model for medical intervention development based on progressive dynamic changes that integrates health technology assessment outcomes with early-stage innovation and indication-specific clinical success rates. Journal of Innovation and Entrepreneurship. 2020;**9**:1. DOI: 10.1186/s13731-019-0111-1